SEXY FEMINISM

A GIRL'S GUIDE TO LOVE, SUCCESS, AND STYLE

JENNIFER KEISHIN ARMSTRONG
and **HEATHER WOOD RUDÚLPH**

SEXY

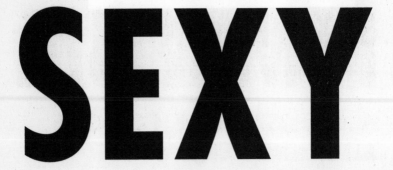

MARINER BOOKS • A MARINER ORIGINAL

FEMINISM

A GIRL'S GUIDE TO LOVE, SUCCESS, AND STYLE

HOUGHTON MIFFLIN HARCOURT • BOSTON • NEW YORK • 2013

For information about permission to reproduce selections from this book,
write to Permissions, Houghton Mifflin Harcourt Publishing Company,
215 Park Avenue South, New York, New York 10003.

www.hmhbooks.com

Library of Congress Cataloging-in-Publication Data
Armstrong, Jennifer Keishin.
Sexy feminism : a girl's guide to love, success, and style / Jennifer
Keishin Armstrong and Heather Wood Rudúlph.
p. cm.
"A Mariner Original."
ISBN 978-0-547-73830-7
1. Self-realization in women. 2. Feminism. 3. Success.
I. Rudúlph, Heather Wood. II. Title.
HQ1206.A735 2013
305.42—dc23
2012040351

Book design by Melissa Lotfy

Printed in the United States of America

DOC 10 9 8 7 6 5 4 3 2 1

Portions of this book first appeared on the authors' website, Sexy Feminist
(www.sexyfeminist.com), and brief portions were reprinted online on The
Huffington Post and AlterNet.

To our mothers,
JoAnn Armstrong and Annette Wood,
who made us the women and
the feminists we are today

CONTENTS

SEXY FEMINISM

A GIRL'S GUIDE TO LOVE, SUCCESS, AND STYLE

OUR OWN FEMINIST JOURNEYS

WE ARE FEMINISTS. But we were not born that way, nor did we have to earn our PhDs in women's studies to get that way (though some serious college study helped). We both started out the most regular of suburban white girls in the 1970s — as if you couldn't tell all of this by our first names. We did not suffer some of the worst injustices of our time: We were not wealthy, but our families had more resources than the vast majority of the world. We were immune to the prejudice gay people our age faced because we were born straight. Our upbringings were almost shockingly mainstream. We both embraced high-school cheerleading without irony, agonized over good grades and boy crushes, and worshipped the likes of Pat Benatar, Madonna, and Cyndi Lauper.

Like our love for those ladies, our feminism evolved — from something cool to reference to something we believed was intrinsic to our lives. You might see a little of yourself in our stories, even if you aren't just like us.

JENNIFER: WORDS GAVE ME THE POWER

My youth in south suburban Chicago, land of winding subdivisions and endless strip malls, did not favor the intellectual or political, though smarts and humor ran deep, and good grades were a priority. My parents and I — I was an only child until age eight — liked food (grilled hamburgers, baked potatoes), music (Simon and Garfunkel, Billy Joel), and baseball (the White Sox, *not* the Cubs). We lived in a brown split-level on a safe cul-de-sac called Forest Court. We liked one another. We acted like *The Brady Bunch*, with fewer kids and less strife. Yes, *that* little strife.

In fact, I consider *both* of my parents to be my first feminist role models. My father worked as a grocery buyer for a chain of stores called Scot Lad Foods, and he was the primary breadwinner. He carried a briefcase in which he kept tantalizing supplies such as yellow legal pads and paper clips, and he let me play office, one of my favorite activities, with his stuff. Even better, I got to visit him at work and sit in his chair, talk on his phone, and doodle on his desk calendar, dreaming of someday having a workplace of my own. I'd watched a lot of *Mary Tyler Moore Show* reruns over the years, and in a twist I'm sure working girl Mary Richards could never have seen coming, I somehow managed to idolize her by idolizing my father.

My mother had a part-time job as a substitute teacher, though she mostly stayed at home to raise me. She served as a best friend as much as a mother, and we shared the same taste in pop music and clothing. I wanted to be her *and* my father at the same time. What a lucky kid.

Of course, traditional gender roles permeated our home life. When Dad came home from a long day at the office and noticed I was wearing something new, he'd say, "That's pretty. Where'd you get that?" And I would answer, "Mom bought it for me." This inspired chuckles from my parents, but only later did I figure out why — it was *Dad* who earned the money, Mom who spent it. Even so, my family counteracted those traditional ideas with lots of empowering messages. My grandfather never stopped talking about how I would be the first woman president. (We'll leave aside the fact that he apparently knew we wouldn't be ready for a female president for at least another forty years or so.) My father played catch with me, taught me chess, and shared his love of astronomy with me. My mother insisted on giving me thorough and repeated sex talks, starting when I was in seventh grade, with lessons on everything from birth control to saying no to when to say yes. (My mother's patented method to ensure the child will listen to these talks: Subject her to them in the car; the kid can't escape.)

When my siblings were born — first my brother, when I was eight, then my sister, when I was ten — I became an assistant parent. This gave me an extra sense of authority and bravado that would come in handy later.

Both my parents supported my first feminist fight, though at the time I didn't realize that's what it was: After spending my formative years as a cheerleader for the Oak Forest Flag Football League, I started coaching the younger girls' cheerleading teams when I was about twelve. At that time, the league decided to turn the annual cheerleading competition into an exhibition — that is, they wanted to eliminate the judging aspect and give everyone a nice participation ribbon and a pat on the head for coming. I would have none of that — if the boys, as football players, could handle weekly competition culminating in an end-of-the-season trophy ceremony ranking teams first, second, and third, surely the girls could compete for one night. To me, competition was what made cheerleading a real sport, a sport I happened to love for its combination of performance, dance, and athletic stunts. I argued just that when I went before the league's board to fight for the cheerleaders' competition. I lost, but I was glad I'd fought.

Such early lessons in gender relations sank in without my thinking about them much, because I was, in many respects, fortunate. Though I suffered a minor sexist setback when our junior-high band director told me I had to play the clarinet instead of the drums — those were for boys, he said — I got to do everything else I wanted. I was a cocaptain of my competitive high-school cheerleading team, sports editor of the school newspaper, and an officer in the National Honor Society and on the student council. I fell in love during my senior year with a boy named Dave who treated me as an equal and best friend, with sexual pressure taking a back seat to intimate talks. Life, overall, went smoothly. I had no reason to believe I would ever be treated as anything but equal — and usually as special.

College changed things. At Northwestern University, I fell behind. I no longer sat at the top of the class. I was getting Ds, I hated my dorm, and I had only one real friend: my perfectly coiffed, well-off, effortlessly successful roommate. Dave broke up with me out of the blue, leaving me to fend for myself among fraternity boys who wanted me to come back to their rooms and who had no interest in hearing my patented "I'm not ready for sex and I hope you'll respect that" talk that had worked just fine on high-school boys. I no longer led anything, I wasn't on any teams or councils, I didn't know what I wanted to do or who I wanted to be, and my roommate made everything look easy — it all brought on massive insecurity. Women's studies classes, however, started to help turn things around. Recognizing my mother's and grandmother's lives — and everything about them I didn't want — in Betty Friedan's *The Feminine Mystique*, I felt like a magic spell had lifted that fate from my shoulders. Simone de Beauvoir seemed to be explaining, well, *everything* in *The Second Sex*. "One is not born, but rather becomes, a woman."

Of course. That's what was happening to me at that moment, and had been for a while — I just hadn't noticed, because life had previously been so kind to me. Now I saw all the messages telling me *You cannot compete; you must not have sex; you must be sexy; you must be sweet.* Womanhood was my problem, in a nutshell. I had become a woman, and I was pissed about it. I did what I could. I read every classic feminist text I could find. I volunteered to be a sexual-assault-prevention educator. (How sad that those were even needed, and that they still are, perhaps more than ever.) I ranted enough about the world's inequalities that my mother admonished me for being "too feminist," which felt like some kind of victory.

Dave came out of the closet, which explained why our high-school relationship had been so romantic — which is to say, so loving but lacking in sexual pressure. Now I was worked up about gay rights, too — I hated the things people said to him as much as I hated the fact that the only love of his life he could marry legally was me, the person with whom he wanted to share lots of things but not sex or marriage.

How had the world become so unjust?

That activist fire dimmed a bit once the real world took hold. I fell in love with a boy in college, and when I graduated, I decided to follow him to Southern California, where he was serving in the U.S. Navy. I became a newspaper reporter, and writing three stories a day about mall plans and petty thefts and county fairs left little time for worrying about empowerment. Not to mention that women had overrun at least the lower ranks of the media business, giving my small world an "oh, good, we're done with that" feeling about feminism. I was more worried about maintaining the rather trying relationship with my boyfriend. It soon became clear that because he was a military man, I was the one who had to bend her life to accommodate the typical early-twenties on-again-off-again liaison. I thought that was what you did to get the brass ring — or, more specifically, the diamond ring — of marriage. You worked at it. You compromised.

This proved true, in a way: We eventually moved to New York, bought a condo together, and got engaged. I started working in magazines, and that's when inequalities began to feel prominent again in my life. I got a job at *Entertainment Weekly*. Its staff was heavy on smart, empowered women, but the industry I was now covering was problematic: Movies and television are not kind to women, particularly women over thirty or those with any discernible physical flaws. It depressed me enough — staring at and meeting freakishly perfect-looking actresses day after day — that I considered going to work at another magazine. But where would I go? To a women's magazine so I could spend my days telling readers how to put on eye shadow and please their men, as if those were the only important things in life? No, thank you. I knew I wanted to stay in the media, and I loved the idea of addressing issues of womanhood, but the way most mainstream women's magazines worked turned me off. And I had an otherwise dream gig at *Entertainment Weekly*, where at least, I figured, I could use my platform to critique the ways pop culture presented women.

Around this same time, I canceled my wedding, even though I had spent a decade dreaming of nothing but marrying the man who was then my fiancé. Things began to unravel when he started planning our life together — a house in suburban New Jersey, a dog, and kids were in his vision of the immediate future, and he simply assumed I wanted the same. It wasn't until he told me this that I knew I definitely *didn't* want it, the way you're not sure what you want to eat for dinner but know it's definitely not Chinese when your dining companion suggests it. I realized, with the same clarity that I know I hate beef chop suey, that I wanted something other than that life in the suburbs raising kids, the life my mother had accepted without question when she married my father, *her* college sweetheart. Nothing against my parents or the suburbs or marriage or kids — I just wanted to take advantage of the choices now afforded to thirty-year-old women, choices feminism gave me.

I *could* enjoy being single. I *could* focus on being a writer, which was what I now knew I wanted more than anything in life.

I *could* live on my own. I also wanted to make my own money and decisions, something that just wasn't built into the DNA of my relationship with my fiancé. He'd always assumed — dare I say it? — the patriarchal role in our partnership, and up to that point, I'd mindlessly let him. Now I saw it clearly, and I couldn't live with it. I didn't know yet how feminist this epiphany was. I just longed for a bigger life.

HEATHER: IMAGINATION + ENCOURAGEMENT = FEMINIST POWER

I grew up in California, the second of six children born to hippies. I used to use this fact as a punch line when talking about my parents. Usually, it came after I disclosed my full name: Heather Spring Wood. Only tree-hugging flower children could come up with that, right? I eventually realized that the hippie ideology meant more than long hair (Dad's ponytail was epic) and an insistence on an organic vegan diet (not particularly yummy to a young child). It was a political statement. Being a hippie in the 1970s and 1980s meant eschewing materialism, embracing unity, and streamlining your life. Much of our food came from the garden and chicken coop that took up most of the backyard. Clothing was handed down, and shiny new toys were scarce. Instead, my mother — who stayed home with us kids while my dad finished school and started a chiropractic practice — let us run wild outside and entertained us by dancing and singing along to her favorite records by the Beatles, Joni Mitchell, and Fleetwood Mac — or, more often than not, just making up her own songs on the fly. It was the perfect environment to cultivate a vivid imagination.

My dad eventually cut his hair, our diet went mainstream, and we got the toys we begged for. It's a challenge to maintain a political, restrictive lifestyle when you have six children who want, want, want! I admire my parents for doing it as long as they did, even if I hated the grainy soy milk and ill-fitting clothes. I credit this upbringing for instilling the hippie-centric values (now a compliment, not a joke) I practice to this day: conscious eating, environmental activism, and feminism.

My parents may have been cast in traditional roles — my father the breadwinner, my mother the caretaker — but this setup was never idealized. Both parents encouraged my siblings and me (just girls for the first six years) to set goals, take risks, and dream of careers. They pushed us to be self-sufficient and accountable. As a big sister, I was often left to care for my younger siblings and lead by example. This gave me a confidence I had perhaps not yet earned. Whenever I faltered, I looked to my early role models for empowerment. If Madonna, Debbie Gibson, and Cyndi Lauper could be superstars, I could do anything, too. My path was decidedly less pop, though. I found my niche as a writer after joining my high-school newspaper, but I didn't know it was my niche until my (female) adviser praised and encouraged me in a way that only my parents had done previously. Not to devalue my parents' important, influential affection, but emotional cheerleading and unadulterated support seem more real when they're not coming from the people who made you.

Ms. Noguchi (decidedly a *Ms.*) was one of my first feminist role models. She made me want to be not just a writer but also a leader. She ruled our rowdy newsroom with wit and discipline. In that environment, the girls seemed to thrive — most of the top editing jobs were filled by my female classmates. She encouraged me to apply for internships and scholarships others had deemed "too competitive" for me (something a male adviser told me on more than one occasion) and cheered on my "leap first, ask questions later" ambition. She knew it would force me to learn some tough lessons along the way (indeed, Ms. Noguchi, indeed), but she saw a spark and didn't want to put it out before the fire could ignite. I was becoming a feminist even if I didn't understand what that was yet.

As I think of all the formative moments in my life, I realize that strong women are the constant. My hard-ass journalism professor at Syracuse University made more than one student cry with her unwavering expectation of excellence (you don't win two Pulitzers without it). When it was my time for tears, she didn't change the first grade of C I'd *ever* seen but instead nurtured my desire to *earn* the A. My first women's studies professor wouldn't pass a student if she didn't commit to part-time volunteerism for at least a year — we had to sign contracts and everything. For a time-starved undergrad, taking on another task seemed impossible, and many dropped the class, but seeing the course through made me realize how important it was (and is) to give to others, always. The news editor at my very first newspaper internship took a red pen to every story I turned in, pointing out lazy sentences and lecturing me (hard) for any factual error. At the time, I thought she hated me; now I know she cared enough to make me remember, learn from, and never repeat my mistakes — an invaluable lesson for me as a journalist and as a person. These strong women reiterated for me the lessons from my parents: Believe in yourself and *be* yourself.

OUR FEMINIST MEET-CUTE

Jennifer and I met when we were both on a journey to find — and become — our true selves. We met when both of our lives were in apparent disarray: we had just lost the men in them. Jennifer had recently broken up with her fiancé, and I had just moved to New York City and left behind a ten-year relationship. A mutual friend recommended I connect with Jennifer because she thought we would click. What an understatement. We bonded first over broken hearts but quickly moved on to a shared passion to do something bigger than the traditional framework of our lives had outlined for us. In a way, we answered each other's need to become a feminist activist.

On our first "date" we went to see, appropriately, *Bend It Like Beckham*, a story of female soccer players and friendship. Afterward, we agreed we hated current women's magazines and wished we had our own publication for which to write, one that would print stories on things we cared about. *Bust* was just emerging as a more modern *Ms.* (and note: swoon!), but the newsstand was dominated by women's self-help magazines — the kinds that tell women how to do everything they already know how to do and how to fix everything that isn't broken. Don't get me wrong: we both loved fashion, makeup, entertainment, and sex. But if we must write about makeup and fashion, we reasoned, couldn't we write about the ways they both empower and restrict us? Wasn't there a lot to be said about how pop culture treats women? Shouldn't someone be writing more in depth and frankly about women's sex lives? Where was all the real information in women's media?

Buzzed on indignation and too much caffeine one Sunday afternoon, we decided to launch a website that did all of that. SirensMag.com went live in January 2006. We learned to run our own business by making lots of mistakes. We found our voices as writers and as feminists. The more we spoke our own truths and allowed other women to do the same as contributors, the more we realized our site wasn't just an alternative online women's magazine, as we'd originally marketed it, but a feminist community.

We relaunched as SexyFeminist.com in 2011 to reflect our now-specific brand of feminism, one that, above all else, owns the oft-maligned word *feminist* and aims to show young women how fun, empowering, and, yes, sexy it is to fight for women's rights and choices. This book grew out of that. We want to help other women find their own feminism, just as we found ours.

We set out on a mission to change publishing, and we changed ourselves instead. And that's what feminism is about: regular people turning themselves into activists through the power of their own thinking.

ONE

WHY FEMINISM IS SEXY

W E'RE HERE TO detonate, once and for all, those pervasive myths about feminism. You know, that it wrecks homes and happiness, that it hates men and sex and anything pretty, that it's a general drag.

Feminism, even in its most classical form, has never aimed to do any of that, but it makes sense that it got mixed up in such ideas. It's a huge movement that's evolved over many decades and split into many factions, although they all have the same aim: equal rights for women. At times, this has meant women leaving their husbands when they realized they wanted more from their lives, demanding equal pay, or telling their spouses to wash their own damn dishes. Sometimes the fight for equality has required flouting beauty standards to make a statement about their silliness —

hence the stereotypical feminist who eschews armpit-shaving and makeup-wearing. The basic idea of equality for women has also spawned more radical ideas. Some splinter feminist groups have, for instance, recommended withdrawing from patriarchal society and establishing entirely new female-run subcultures, ruled out any sex with men as inherently fraught with inequality, and declared lesbianism the only logical orientation for a decent feminist.

Feminism is mostly past this by now, but in mainstream society, the movement's image as a buzzkill lingers, making it a tough sell even for many of the ambitious young women who have benefited from it. With this book, we hope to dispel those negative ideas about feminism once and for all, but, more important, we hope to give any woman with the slightest desire for female empowerment the tools to bring feminist ideals into her everyday life.

We like Gloria Steinem's take on the word *feminist*: "the belief in the full social, economic, and political equality of women and men. I would just add 'and doing something about it.' And when you look at the effects of that simple statement, it's quite a transformation." We couldn't agree more. We see it like this. Step 1: Call yourself a proud *feminist*. Step 2: Live up to the word. Seems like a pretty easy first step, but the F-word has long been a stumbling block for the movement. It was first used in the 1870s in France to describe women agitating for change. By the time it showed up in the English language, in the 1890s, the term had already become derogatory. Or at least it was meant to be when the *UK Daily News* warned its readers of a dangerous new trend, "what our Paris Correspondent describes as a 'Feminist' group." Even the more benign-sounding movement for "votes for women" got a bad rap when Queen Victoria called it a "mad, wicked folly." About the same time that *feminism* officially became a word in the *Oxford English Dictionary*, in 1894, the women's suffrage movement, commonly considered the first wave of feminism, was heating up. American women got the vote in 1920, and things died down until the second wave — the women's lib movement of the '60s and '70s, which brought us the Equal Rights Amendment, *Roe v. Wade*, *Ms.* magazine, and a barrage of other political, sexual, and social breakthroughs. During that time, the word *feminism* took on the specific negative connotations that continue to plague it today (see above lesbian separatist movements and unshaven armpits).

Feminism's Waves, a Brief History

First Wave: The late nineteenth- and early-twentieth-century activists who fought, primarily in the United States, the United Kingdom, Canada, and the Netherlands, for legal equality for women — specifically, for women's right to vote.

Second Wave: Often thought of by modern young women as *the* feminist movement, this was a period of activity that peaked in the 1970s but lasted, arguably, through the 1980s. This massive push for equality gave us Gloria Steinem and *Ms.* magazine; greater sexual freedom and reproductive rights; awareness of child care, equal wages, sexual harassment, and sexual assault as major issues; and, alas, the failed Equal Rights Amendment.

Third Wave: From the late 1980s onward, a new generation of feminists took over and responded to the second wave's gains, losses, and weaknesses. Sex positivity, more diverse cultural awareness, and critiquing and contributing to pop culture (Riot Grrrl!) became its hallmarks.

Fourth Wave and Beyond: Perhaps beginning right now, this new movement within the movement may resist labels but most definitely will include even greater media awareness, cultural and sexual diversity, and lots and lots of blogs.

The "I'm not a feminist, but . . ." problem spread during the 1980s backlash and persists today, and we'd love to see that stop. But *feminist* is just a word, you might say — why is it so important? Given the choice between living feminist principles and calling ourselves feminists, of course we'd choose the former. But we don't think there should have to be a choice. To distance yourself from the word is to imply there's something wrong with feminism and/or feminists, an implication that leads to the continued denigration of the cause itself. Ladies, if we can reclaim words like *slut* and *bitch*, using them, Riot Grrrl–style, to denote power instead of degradation, we can reclaim the word *feminist*.

Of course, calling yourself a feminist doesn't give you a free pass to do whatever you want in the name of your personal liberation, as many prominent women and submovements claim. You know: "Plastic surgery is my right as a feminist. If it makes me feel good, I should do it because I'm a woman and also all that beauty advertising keeps telling me that 'I'm worth it.'" Or "Being on the cover of *Maxim* in my underwear is a statement of my sexual empowerment!" Or "I'm totally a feminist even though I'm pro-life and pretty much anti-woman in all my policies, though at least

I quit my job as governor of Alaska so it's not like I can actually make policy anymore." (That one's kind of specific, but you get the idea.)

Yes, Naomi Wolf said that "the enemy is not lipstick, but guilt itself; that we deserve lipstick, if we want it, AND free speech; we deserve to be sexual AND serious — or whatever we please; we are entitled to wear cowboy boots to our own revolution." We think she's right about all of that. But we don't think she meant every single fun female act is inherently feminist just because it feels freeing.

As far as we're concerned, your actions affect the world and the women around you whether or not you're famous, and being a feminist means taking that responsibility seriously in every aspect of your life, from choosing eye shadow to flirting to fighting for birth control rights. Even the busiest modern professional woman can make room for feminism in her life, and in fact, we think she's in a unique position to do so — with her votes, her dollars, and her actions. In this book, we'll give you some ideas about how to do that like a true Sexy Feminist. We'll also give you resources so you can look further into a variety of feminist-minded causes, whether that means picking up some of the foundational books of modern feminism or getting involved with your local Planned Parenthood.

If you need a reason to call yourself a feminist, we'll give you a few. For starters, feminism makes all of our lives better, in every possible way, period; smiling, feeling good, and occasional indulgences are more than welcome. Second-wave feminists — think Steinem and *The Feminine Mystique* author Betty Friedan — came across as quite serious, and for good reason. They needed to demand that the world take them seriously, and they effected major change by doing so. Their even more radical cohorts did us some major good too. Only when activists make extreme arguments do movements get the attention they need, and the progress they deserve, by pulling the debate farther over to their side. Many strands of what's now recognized as the third wave swung too far the other way, though, causing commentators to scoff at "do-me" feminists and "bimbo" feminists who seemed to advocate flaunting one's body for empowerment and sleeping one's way to liberation. As the movement enters what could become the fourth wave, even those of us who proudly identify ourselves as feminists are stuck between second- and third-wave approaches.

We think our second-wave predecessors were right: the personal couldn't be more political than it is in this movement, and that's important to remember. But we also think the third-wavers who appreciate pretty things, love playing with beauty products, express themselves through fashion, adore having partners to love, celebrate their sexuality, and even kind of dig some cooking and keeping house are right too. In this guide, we offer a starting point for reconciling those approaches by supporting responsible, feminist companies; thinking through the broader implications of your consumption, conversation, and bedroom and boardroom decisions; and, above all, supporting other women. For us, philosopher Immanuel Kant's categorical imperative is as true for issues like boob jobs and bikini waxes as it is for anything else: "Act only according to that maxim whereby you can, at the same time, will that it should become a universal law." Put another way: The higher the number of women who get boob jobs, the higher the number of women who will feel pressured to get boob jobs — therefore, getting a boob job is not a feminist act, no matter what Lisbeth Salander does in *The Girl Who Played with Fire*.

As you ponder these issues, we hope you'll become part of the larger movement, if you haven't already. This movement, despite regular "We Don't Need Feminism" headlines, is more critical to our health, wealth, and happiness than ever. But feminism can be poring over makeup and beauty products — if you're into that kind of thing — to find the ones that make you feel good specifically because your buying them empowers female-led businesses. Feminism is about loving your lady parts, whether they're painstakingly (or painfully) groomed or as natural as can be. It's running a marathon because it feels good, not because it burns calories. It's scaling unprecedented career heights and pulling other women up there with you. It's answering the phone when your girlfriend calls at midnight for a pick-me-up and being supportive and honest rather than man-bashing just to make her feel better.

Feminism is also finding the right partners — whatever that means to you — and not tolerating the wrong ones. It is caring for your partners as they do for you. It is the freedom of safe sex and of welcoming children into your life when and if you're ready. It is defining your own sense of style, whether that means miniskirts and stilettos or cargo pants and army boots. It's enjoying — nay, demanding — mind-blowing romps in the sack, and giving in to true love sometimes, naked lust other times.

Of course, feminism is all the things that word traditionally brings to mind as well — rallies for reproductive rights, de Beauvoir and Friedan, *Ms.* and demands for equal pay. (How is equal pay not happening yet?) But you don't have to launch a feminist blog, major in women's studies, or paint a protest sign to bring feminism into your life. In fact, choices you make every day can turn into acts of empowerment, for yourself and for womankind. That's what this book is all about: looking at the history behind and the pros and cons of some of the most common consumption and lifestyle decisions that have been tripwires for feminists. Read the chapters that feel most relevant to you; ponder the questions we pose at the end of each chapter, or, better yet, bring them to your next wine-fueled girls' night for discussion; and then look into ways to deepen your activism, perhaps starting with some of the resources provided at the end of this book.

And please keep in mind that even if every minute of every day of your life isn't explicitly feminist, you needn't eject yourself from the club. We're not here to pile more onto the load of perfectionist pressures women already bear. Do what you can, and then do some more. If you fall off the feminist wagon, just get back on. We'll happily pull you up.

That, ladies, is what being a Sexy Feminist is all about.

Sexy Feminist: Tina Fey

Forget Carrie Bradshaw. When it comes to TV role models, we'll take Tina Fey's harried, sub-sandwich-eating, white-wine-swilling goofball alter ego Liz Lemon any day over a certain well-dressed, man-hungry Manhattanite.

Fey's *30 Rock*, a showbiz-based sitcom about a hard-working TV writer and her awkward life/love shenanigans, gave women a role model who was more relatable — and thus more powerful — than Carrie Bradshaw, the heroine of that feminist mixed bag known as *Sex and the City*. If Carrie is a descendant of *Breakfast at Tiffany's* Holly Golightly, Liz is the spiritual daughter of *Mary Tyler Moore's* Mary Richards. Carrie's wardrobe, killer body, glamorous social life, and inexplicable financial solvency just make us feel bad about our schlubby lives; Liz helps us laugh at our foibles. While both Liz and Carrie have their feminist merits, Liz Lemon represents the woman most of us *truly* feel like in this rushed, complicated new millennium. A woman trying to balance a successful career, various bungled relationships, and an appetite for junk food looks far more familiar to most of us than one who pens sex columns between glamorous parties and four-hundred-dollar-shoe–buying sprees.

Liz Lemon captures the quintessential lady problem of the modern age: the frustration and futility of trying to have it all. The ridiculous nature by which she fails and flails serves as Fey's critique on the expectations placed on educated, ambitious career women everywhere. Tina Fey the woman — a wife and mother in real life — has managed to defy this stereotype, giving her further feminist cred.

Fey proved for a new generation of women that smart is sexy — even when you're wearing glasses! (Baton passed, Lisa Loeb.) You'll see her in sultry clothing on the cover of magazines, but inside, she's likely making fun of that outfit. She lives by the credo that speaking up is better than shutting up, and damn the consequences. Tina Fey at her most feminist is also Tina Fey at her most controversial. When she popped into "Women's News" segments on *SNL*'s "Weekend Update" in 2007 and 2008, Fey celebrated women's accomplishments (Hillary Rodham Clinton's work, the successes of female astronauts) as well as ridiculed their low points (the Pussycat Dolls, celebrity mistresses). During the 2008 presidential primaries, Fey snapped at the sexist talk aimed at Clinton, defending women as the ones who make society work. "Bitches get stuff done!" she railed on *SNL*. And then she coined what may have been the feminist phrase of the decade: "Bitch is the new black."

Feminism has, without a doubt, delivered its share of victories over the past decades. We have more women running for office — and winning — than ever before, and occasionally voters even see them as more than just the female candidates. Feminists have managed at least to keep a watchful eye on our under-fire reproductive rights. Both genders now move more freely than ever between roles. Women outnumber men in college classes and medical schools.

And yet we still have a culture that glorifies a violent, objectifying man named Charlie Sheen. The *New York Times* frets (in a 2011 story) over how the small-town–Texas gang rape of an eleven-year-old girl will affect the lives of the eighteen men and boys involved while also describing the victim's provocative style of dress and lack of adult supervision. Society still pressures women to get married and procreate. Pole dancing is allegedly a valid form of exercise. Magazines and websites run items on whether the calorie count of semen is high enough to cause blowjob-induced weight gain. Many men still find it intimidating, or at least unsexy, when a woman describes herself as a feminist.

Overall, we're still taught to think we're not enough specifically because we are women. As third-wave author Jessica Valenti said in her book *Full Frontal Feminism*, "As different as we all are, there's one thing most young women have in common: We're all brought up to feel like there's something wrong with us. We're too fat. We're dumb. We're too smart. We're not ladylike enough — *stop cursing, chewing with your mouth open, speaking your mind.* We're too slutty. We're not slutty enough."

It's specifically because of these dichotomies that feminism has grown increasingly complicated. Even among people who agree feminism is a good thing, debates rage: Is dressing sexy a sign of liberation or submission to patriarchy? Is marriage sexist? And why shouldn't pole dancing be considered a valid form of exercise? Shouldn't strippers be empowered too? Many women also still associate this F-word with a set of rules that they don't agree with: Hate men; don't shave; and button up your shirt.

Because this movement deals with such close-to-home issues, it has always courted murky questions. Women in the United States fought for decades to gain the vote; they received it in 1920, only to find the battles far from over on issues such as unmarried women's poverty and reproductive rights, all the more relevant during the post-crash economic downturn of the 1930s. Women entered the work force en masse during World War II only to find this meant pulling double duty as employees *and* homemakers. Many found themselves once more imprisoned by their wifely duties during the ultraconservative 1950s, suffering from what Friedan would term the feminine mystique. The sexual revolution of the 1960s gave us the right to free love and orgasms, causing Steinem to opine that "a Liberated Woman was somebody who had sex before marriage and a job afterward." But that liberated attitude paved the way for what Ariel Levy would call female chauvinist pigs — women who objectified themselves so men didn't have to bother. The advertising and entertainment industries continue to co-opt feminism and use its ideas against us, packaging the concepts of women's liberation and girl power and using them to sell us everything from shoes and Botox parties to the Spice Girls and the Pussycat Dolls.

But feminism's many gray areas also leave lots of room for all kinds of women to identify themselves as feminists. College students getting their first taste of women's studies and women working on the frontlines of the movement every day can stand alongside mom bloggers and overworked CEOs, burlesque dancers and makeup artists. Whether every kind of woman — particularly women of color and lesbian, bisexual, or transsexual women — feels included in the movement as it now stands remains a matter of debate. We must, however, make room in the discussion for anyone willing to call herself a feminist and fight for genuine equality.

That's why we've come up with our own sexy, fun, empowering brand of feminism — and why we encourage every woman out there to come up with her own as well. So, yes, that means rules, but they're your own. It doesn't have to mean giving up shaving — or waxing, makeup, high-heeled shoes, short skirts, dates with men, or porn. By making feminism relevant to our daily lives, and resonant with our own unique values, we can save the movement, one woman at a time, and bring it into our fraught twenty-first century.

Women are constantly making decisions that can have far more feminist impact than they realize — in the bedroom, the boardroom, the kitchen, the mall, and the locker room. And in our media-centric world, music, movies, TV, and blogs offer up more room for feminist debate than ever before. Modern women can make as much of a feminist impact by demanding their partners wear condoms or debating the feminist merits of Taylor Swift on a blog message board as they can by supporting NOW or writing a long-form scholarly essay about the insidious nature of patriarchy. Of course the latter two matter. They have always mattered, and they will until the world is equal. But bringing the message into everyday life instead of the same old feminist venues will define today's feminism. Calling yourself a feminist, proudly, because it's a fucking awesome thing to be is one way to do just that. As Gloria Steinem said, "If you don't stand up for yourself politically, no one else will. So we have to use our votes and our dollars and our voices to be engaged and involved in these issues."

You can be a feminist right now. You can start at any moment, altering your life one little decision at a time. It doesn't call for a major upheaval, most likely. It just requires commitment to being more conscious, something you've undoubtedly done before when you've counted calories or flirted methodically or decoded your boyfriend's every move or applied your makeup just like that women's magazine told you to. Except this time, we're asking all of you to do this in the name of women — in the name of your mothers, sisters, friends, coworkers, and, of course, yourselves.

Now it's time for you to find your own sexy feminism.

Some of Our Favorite Sexy Feminists

Suze Orman. The personal finance guru (and author of nine bestsellers, including *Women and Money*) makes financial freedom an achievable goal for women everywhere. Her books serve as wake-up calls for a generation of women who benefited from good educations and no-holds-barred ambitions but then found them-

selves in a consumerism trap and often victimized by financial insti-
tutions. We can think of no better way to empower women than by
giving them power over money.

Supreme Court Justice Sonia Sotomayor. Being the first
Latina justice and only the third female justice in the history of the
United States makes the lady an icon. Rising from a struggling
family in the Bronx to Princeton and then Yale Law? Even better.
On top of all that, she kept her cool — and her sense of humor —
throughout a confirmation process that questioned not her quali-
fications (her lifelong dedication to her career made that pretty
tough), but her sexual orientation and single status. When President Obama swore her in, she credited her greatest role model:
her mother, to whom she often referred as "my life inspiration."
"I stand on the shoulders of countless people, yet there is one ex-
traordinary person who is my life aspiration — that person is my
mother."

Christiane Amanpour. A handful of women have broken
through the glass ceiling of the still-male-dominated TV news business — Barbara Walters, Oprah Winfrey, Katie Couric, Diane Saw-
yer. But few women have exhibited as much brave ambition and
tenacity as Amanpour. Reporting for CNN and ABC, she has been
on the scene of most every major war and humanitarian crisis of
the past two decades, often bringing people's attention to stories
other media outlets ignored. Most impressive is the way she lobs
hardball questions at dictators and world leaders, especially those
guilty of some of the greatest crimes against humanity. She is *kick-
ass* personified.

Shonda Rhimes. The *Grey's Anatomy* creator and executive
producer is a black woman playing what's traditionally — and still

overwhelmingly — a white man's game. But she's not playing it *like a white man* so she can fit in. In fact, she pioneered the concept of colorblind casting when she assembled the stunning ensemble of the doctor drama that became a national obsession. She demanded to see actors of all colors for all the roles, picked the best ones for the job — and, lo and behold, she had not only the most diverse cast on television but also one of the most talented. On top of that, she presents a subversively feminist utopia on *Grey's* as well as another show of hers, *Private Practice.* Here, men and women have equality without question — if anyone is objectified, it's the men. Women can have any job and act any way they want — yes, that means being inspirational figures like world-class surgeons and enviable lesbian couples, but it also means being drinkers, whiners, bitches, and unapologetic sleep-arounders. We'd happily check into Seattle Grace, even with all the angst that seems to ensue.

Portia de Rossi and Ellen DeGeneres. These two gorgeous, talented ladies send an important message as the most mainstream lesbian power couple ever. The sexy, smart, funny, out-and-proud pair makes gay marriage a more accessible concept for the masses. Portia looks like a straight man's fantasy girl — tall and blond, with exotic features and an accent to boot — but she defends gay rights every chance she gets and isn't afraid to expose the ugliness in her own life to help others. Her 2010 memoir, *Unbearable Lightness: A Story of Loss and Gain,* chronicled her near-lifelong battle with eating disorders. When she accepts who she is — even though her life is contrary to the popular opinion of what's normal — she finds peace and happiness, a feminist message for the masses.

Ellen sacrificed a career to live her truth and became one of America's national treasures in the process. Her 1990s sitcom, *Ellen,* was canceled after she came out and demanded that her character do the same. Today, she's the closest thing we've got to a new Oprah with her Emmy-winning eponymous talk show. A gay woman holding the heartstrings of Middle America is rivaled in significance only by a black woman running her own TV network. And let's talk about significant media presence: DeGeneres's omnipresent Cover Girl ads are a small but critical step toward reforming the way the media depicts beauty. Now that's sexy feminism.

TWO

OUR POOR VAGINAS

WHEN A *COSMO* HEADLINE promises to help readers get a "healthy, sexy vagina," you know we've gone wrong somewhere. Here, all this time, we thought if we had just one inch of sexy on ourselves, it resided in *our sex organs*. We figured maybe, just maybe, the place where their penises go might turn men on. We thought that perhaps the millions who paused their VHS tapes of the 1992 movie *Basic Instinct* at a certain moment — when Sharon Stone uncrosses her legs for all the world to see a flash of her goods — were already predisposed to like pussy. (Then again, that *is* a hot white minidress she wears; maybe they were just appreciating the simplicity of the design.) What we're saying is we didn't realize it could be such a chore to sex up the part of us that performs the sex.

Oops, take that back: We *did* realize it. We've realized it since the late '90s, when suddenly it wasn't just porn stars who found it necessary to hire a lady to pour hot wax onto their genitals and then rip it *allll* off to, you know, keep things tidy down there. Organized. *Sexy*. In fact, a startling number of us were complicit in this painful trend — known by the seductive term *Brazilian bikini wax* — especially given that, unlike porn stars and swimsuit models, most of us couldn't even claim it as a tax write-off. Among women in American cities, this procedure has even become the norm, as routine as a manicure-pedicure or highlights, more routine than a dentist appointment. It is no mere biannual affair, after all. Keeping your honeypot sexy takes dedication, darling.

The question: Why do we do this? And the corollary: Does every rip of the wax take a little bit of our feminism with it?

To figure that out, it's worth looking at bikini waxing's history. The practice of hair removal dates back to 3000 B.C. and the advent of razors, but the practice of waxing as we know it crept into America in the 1950s as bathing-suit bottoms advanced upward, though in its first half century or so of existence, it involved taking just the hair that extended beyond the panty line — the procedure now known as the traditional or basic bikini wax. Models and others whose careers depended on how they looked in teeny scraps of clothing accepted it as an occupational hazard by the 1970s. Arnold Schwarzenegger joked in 2003 that choosing to run for governor of California was the hardest decision he'd ever made except for when he'd decided to get a bikini wax in 1978.

It was in 1994 that Brazilians hit U.S. shores. They washed up, as so many things do, in Manhattan. The J. Sisters, an ingenious group of seven Brazilian-immigrant siblings, introduced trend-crazed females to what they said was all the rage in their native country. "In Brazil, waxing is part of our culture because bikinis are so small," Jonice Padilha explains on their website. "We thought it was an important service to add because personal care is no longer a luxury, it's a necessity."

Such words — *personal care, luxury, necessity, small* — sound like a dare to appearance-obsessed celebrities weighed down by too much money. By 1999, Gwyneth Paltrow, Kirstie Alley, and Jennifer Grey were singing the J. Sisters' praises. *You've changed my life!* Paltrow signed a photo to the J. Sisters that hangs on their salon wall.

But sixty to a hundred dollars a month may have seemed a little steep to the non-celebrities among us, even for a life-changing experience. It was the porn that finally got to us and that made Brazilian waxes such a postmillennial phenomenon. Women weren't as prone as men to hitting the back room of the local Video King just to check out other ladies' equipment, but it's possible we might have sometimes wandered over to the porn department at Google. Meanwhile, lad mags like *Maxim* and *Gear* rose to prominence, stealing buzz from stalwarts such as *GQ* and *Esquire* by mainstreaming a soft-porn aesthetic even on grocery-store magazine racks. (*Maxim* shot to an impressive 2.2-million-reader circulation, almost three times that of *GQ*.) Jenna Jameson and other adult-film stars became household names; Jameson's 2004 memoir with the self-helpy title *How to Make Love Like a Porn Star* turned into a mega-bestseller — the public wanted to know exactly that. And what we found, the more we looked at porn, was that there was not a female pubic hair in sight. And then many of us thought: *If guys like porn and I want to have sex*

with men, it just seems logical that I should not have pubic hair.
Not the most feminist thought, of course, but that's what happens
when we're bombarded with certain images. Plus, sex clouds one's
thinking sometimes.

This trend gained in popularity, even though the embarrassment of getting a bikini wax could be even more painful than the
physical ripping was. It became a routine occurrence to pick your
legs up over your head, approaching yoga's plow position, and/or
turn over on your side and spread your cheeks for the nice lady
making you pretty. It became normal to have conversations with
salon professionals about whether you wanted a postage stamp
of hair (sometimes dubbed a French wax), even less (sometimes
called a Mediterranean), or nothing (the classic Brazilian). A note:
Since most major spas now just call a beyond-basic wax a Brazilian and ask you when you get there how much hair to leave, we'll
use that term here for any sort of wax that gets your crotch cam-
era-ready. (And for those who are too afraid to ask: We're talking
bare, from front to labia to back.) It's best that everyone knows what
we're talking about here before we proceed.

WAXING TAKES AMERICA

Many of us, for obvious reasons, had some reservations about the
process when waxing first started showing up on salon price lists
throughout the country. That is, until pop culture intervened. *Sex
and the City* took the first step, as was often the case with trends
that cropped up during its years on the air, in a September 2000
episode in which hapless sex columnist Carrie Bradshaw gets a
Brazilian while vacationing in Los Angeles. Carrie didn't look like

she was having a lot of fun during the ordeal, but let's face it — at that time, many women wanted to do whatever Carrie did, even things that looked torturous, like wearing dangerously high heels and dating Mr. Big. *Sex and the City* validated waxing as a standard practice even as it hinted at its painful underpinning — its not-so-feminist side. Now waxing wasn't just a way to emulate porn stars and conform to patriarchal beauty standards. It was a way to emulate a female pop-culture icon with whom the word *empowered* was often connected.

By the time the first decade of the millennium was winding down, Brazilians were a standard offering on the price list of any spa worth visiting. (And many that weren't worth visiting: For the love of Carrie Bradshaw, who gets twenty-two-dollar acrylics and thirty-dollar Brazilians in the same establishment? When it comes to this procedure, please, ladies, do not bargain-hunt.) We knew it had reached the masses when, in 2009, suburban-mom staple *The View* featured a segment in which cohost Sherri Shepherd got a wax. (It bore a stunning resemblance to the Carrie sequence nine years earlier, with a bonus line: "This is worse than having a baby!") Then even mainstream prime-time hit *Grey's Anatomy* addressed waxes as de rigueur for a third date during a 2010 episode. Preparing the surgical field, the sexy TV doctors called it with a wink. The sensible, inexperienced-with-dating Dr. Miranda Bailey balked at the ridiculousness of it all. "She held up two postage stamps and asked if I was looking for the forty-four-cent or the three," she complained, rattled from her virgin visit to the waxer, but the implication was clear. Silly Miranda. *Everyone* knows you need to pare it all down to a landing strip if you're up to the third date.

THE UPSIDE

Waxing has become such an ingrained habit — like eyebrow-plucking or cuticle-cutting — that many of us have grown to *like* regular bikini waxes, so much so that we get them even when no one but our waxers will see those particular parts of us for the near future. Are we brainwashed, or do we have good reason? Well, for starters, waxes do make you feel clean. They appeal to that OCD side so many of us have when it comes to appearance; they keep things squared away, like a haircut or a facial. We shave our armpits and our legs — why not our pubic hair too? The beach argument — the original reason for modern bikini waxes — holds up. Even some of the most dedicated feminists can get behind the idea of not displaying one's pubes when parading the rest of oneself in the name

Vagina Moments in Pop-Culture History

1992: Sharon Stone flashes the world in *Basic Instinct*

2000: Bikini waxes featured on an episode of *Sex and the City* spark water-cooler debates

2006: *Grey's Anatomy* popularizes use of the term *va-jay-jay* (Oprah then runs with it and makes it mainstream)

2006: Britney Spears flashes the world in paparazzi pics

2010: Via an oft-quoted interview, Jennifer Love Hewitt unleashes the vajazzling trend ("the act of applying glitter and jewels to a woman's nether regions for aesthetic purposes," according to vajazzling.com) on the unsuspecting world of summer. That's just basic manners. And waxing can be considered an improvement, of sorts, over 1980s hair-removal methods such as Nair (there's a reason that chemical cocktail makes your hair fall out — it's toxic!) and the Epilady (ouch!). Even good old-fashioned shaving can leave a mess of ingrown hairs at best and cuts at worst. If you can take a blade to your nether regions, why not wax?

Most women's-health experts agree bikini waxes cause no harm, provided they're done by a safe, clean, and reputable salon (again, ladies, no bikini waxes in strip-mall nail salons, please!). Some doctors say pubic hair might provide some minor protective functions, though the need for those functions has lessened in our age of, you know, clothing and underwear. In fact, no modern-day woman *needs* pubic hair for anything. It's just a vestige of our more animalistic days, when nature thought it would be a good idea to keep bacteria out and keep the odors alluring to cavemen in.

And that brings us to the real issue here. Let's just say it: we do it for sex. Youngest J. Sister, Jonice, said it best (if very Brazilian) when she told the *New York Observer*: "Makes you sexy. Makes you fashion. When I don't have my bikini wax, I don't feel like to have sex with my husband. I feel dirty. And even himself say, 'Try a bikini wax!' I feel free. I feel clean." It's simple physics: we can feel more without the bush in the way. Of *course* the standard-issue labia have worked just fine since the beginning of humanity. There's no real reason to mess with the area, and you'll have satisfying sex without a wax. (Any partner who tells you otherwise can get his or her share elsewhere.) However, with less hair in the way, the labia and the all-important clitoris are closer to the action, easy to find, and unimpeded. With a wax, a woman's junk is almost as accessible as, yes, a man's. This isn't about oppression and pornification; it's about logistics. Though we'd also encourage anyone planning to have sex with a woman to take some time to look at a diagram of female anatomy and learn where everything is, pubic hair or none.

THE OTHER SIDE

The problem, of course, is that waxing can slip easily from conscious grooming choice into vulva hatred and abuse. For starters, waxing feels a little like the more painful and expensive cousin of douching. Back in the 1970s and '80s, cleaning out the vagina with a little Summer's Eve was all the rage — commercials featuring ladies in gauzy dresses convinced us that all vaginas were cesspools of disgustingness that could be turned into meadows and walks on the beach with the right product. Later, we found out douching not only wasn't necessary but could cause pelvic inflammatory disease — which, besides being painful, can lead to ectopic pregnancy and sterility. These days, the waxing industry has convinced us that making the vagina "better" is worth eighty dollars a month and the kind of pain that requires special breathing exercises to endure. (Sample rave review on Yelp.com for a salon's waxing procedure: "I truly hate getting bikini waxes, but after my experience today I will hate them a little less." This is worth a five-star rating on a site where citizen reviewers have been known to rant that a restaurant should be torn down if the hostess kept them waiting five extra minutes or the waiter brought them lukewarm coffee.)–

Feminist Confessions: Waxing That Caused Embarrassment, Feminist Guilt, and (Eventually) Feeling Okay with Going Bare

The first time I got a Brazilian bikini wax my then boyfriend laughed — not exactly the afterglow I was expecting. We had been dating for many years and during this phase we were in a long-distance relationship. So for one of his visits I thought I'd surprise him with something sexy and new. After all, women's magazines, female-targeted TV shows, and even my friends were hinting at the power of the Brazilian. So I went out and got myself some designer pubic hair.

And he laughed.

What I learned from this hairy little incident is the importance of talking — and listening — to your partner. My guy, who's now my husband, often calls himself a man of the '70s, so *of course* he laughed; he wanted Pam Grier, not Pam Anderson. It was definitely a relief to know he didn't *expect* such meticulous grooming. But I kept waxing anyway; I learned that personal grooming was personal, and if I liked it, it was my choice. And I did like it; still do. Yes, it's clean, it's easy to maintain, it banishes ingrown hairs (a nasty problem for my very fair-skinned self), and it increases sensitivity during sex. But mostly I just like being taken care of down there. It's one less thing to worry about in the ongoing maintenance routine that is a woman's life. This convenience factor is so key that I even employed the waxer days before giving birth (vaginally) to my son. Trust me, this alleviated *a lot* of unwanted maintenance drama (grooming a vagina still recovering from birth trauma

= not fun) in the days following. And now that I'm a busy mom, waxing is an aesthetic indulgence that saves me time.

Truth be told and understood: Waxing hurts like a son of a bitch. The pain is minimal if I manage to keep my monthly appointments, but let just one slip and I'm back to cursing my very kind and skilled aesthetician. So is it worth it? For me, yes. I am a shout-from-the-rooftops feminist and I know using hot wax to rip my genital hair from its place is not necessarily an inherently feminist act. But I feel just a little empowered knowing that I am making this decision for myself. I'm not doing it because I think guys like it (which is often the assumption behind many women's choice to get Brazilians, although it's not always the reality). My guy wishes I had *more* pubic hair (I've adopted a somewhere-between-bare-and-bush style — hey, relationships are about compromise!), and I turn into a blushing, giggling idiot if I see porn, so I certainly don't idolize its look. For me, waxing is just an informed, agonized-over, resolute choice that I'm making about *my* lady business. And I'm okay with it.

— *Heather Wood Rudúlph*

Waxing is also a practice that, if done by the wrong aesthetician, can lead to chafing, bruising, and worse. In 2009, after two women were hospitalized with waxing-related infections in New Jersey, the state considered banning the service altogether. Even if there are no severe complications from the procedure, burns and cuts can result, not to mention that skin can come off with the wax. Waxing isn't even close to being on par with the travesty of, say, female genital mutilation or foot binding — although waxing critics have compared it to both — but it's a little step closer to those when it's done cheaply and brutally.

There's also the matter of competing with porn stars, a battle that doesn't end with intimate-hair care. Some women (including one of the authors here, in a previous life known as her twenties) start getting Brazilians at the request of their Internet-porn-raised Generation X and Y boyfriends. There's no doubt many men appreciate it. Here's one quoted in the Canadian website Slice's "Ask a Guy" column: "A Brazilian wax brings out fantasies that a lot of mature men would not want to talk about because they may be looked upon as sick perverts. So, yeah, get the full Brazilian wax." But as one waxer told us, "Women are requesting the Brazilian as if it were a haircut style. I tell them they should send their guys in here for a chest wax for a little context to their demands — Brazilians are no joke." Amen.

Still, so many women line up to do it, terrified they might lose out to other women who have outgroomed them. The potential for pain does not deter women from following one another into the salon. As one blogger at DivineCaroline.com wrote while preparing to get her first wax: "For years, I've heard horror stories of the Brazilian bikini wax. Getting down on all fours, raising a leg like a dog peeing on a tree, spreading my butt cheeks to allow a complete stranger to apply hot wax in the most private crevices of my body . . . these didn't seem like things I needed to rush out and experience (at least not in public). Friends of mine — amazing women with high pain tolerances who'd squeezed 10-pound babies out of a 10-centimeter hole — told me they'd cried from the pain of a Brazilian. What was I doing?"

And there's the message we're sending to ourselves — and to

men — that what we were born with isn't good enough as it is, another idea whose implications are not about to stop at the bikini line. As that "Ask a Guy" respondent alluded to, we also happen to be making ourselves look like ten-year-old girls, which is disturbing, to say the least. Isn't one of the most distinctive features of pubic hair the fact that it shows up at puberty, making it one of the most reliable signs of sexual maturity?

Hell, even our language has altered to reflect our societal confusion about women's private parts. In this book, we've chosen to refer to the entire lady business as a vagina, as most women's media now do. (See the *Cosmo* cover line at the beginning of this chapter.) But technically, *vagina* refers to the inner canal of the female reproductive system; the outer parts that get waxed are the labia. Let's just say you'd never catch a man confusing his penis with his testicles.

AFTER THE BRAZILIAN: VAGINAS GONE WILD

Another problem with the world going Brazilian: it has opened the floodgates to far more egregious vagina-altering trends. With bare vaginas as the norm, how do you add that extra something to mark a special occasion? Why, you vajazzle! Yes, women get their crotches bedazzled by trained professionals, who stick tiny adhesive sparkles on their hair-free parts. "After a breakup, a friend of mine Swarovski crystalled my, um, precious lady," actress Jennifer Love Hewitt told George Lopez on his talk show in January 2010. "It shined like a disco ball." What had been a (weird) niche market exploded into a buzzy trend. Even those of us who wax rolled our eyes. What would be next?

Why, glad you asked! Labial plastic surgery took off in 2006, as Brazilian waxing became the norm and women could see supposed imperfections. After that came vaginal rejuvenation, which uses laser treatments to tighten the vagina. (Please note: laser treatments are not as quick and painless and *Star Wars*–like as they sound; see our chapter on cosmetic surgery for more.) "Our mission is to empower women with knowledge, choice and alternatives," says the website of Strax Rejuvenation. "In one of our patient surveys, women were asked: do women want to be loose or relaxed or do women want to be tight? Women answered 100 percent — women want to be tight." Tight . . . *and* virginal: Plastic surgeons also now push re-hymenization, an extra-special-occasion procedure that allows you to give your loved one your virginity all over again. It's hard to avoid making the connection between the tightening procedures and the infantilization argument against Brazilian waxing.

It turns out, however, that even *actual* young girls could use some improvement, according to some shady spas now giving preteen girls bikini waxes. "For waxing, 12 years old is the 'new normal,'" Philadelphia aesthetician Melanie Engle told the *Today* show's website. Sure, girls develop ever younger these days, but how necessary could this be? One New York salon even goes so far as to advertise special rates for "virgin" waxing. "Virgin hair can be waxed so successfully that growth can be permanently stopped in just two to six sessions," explains the website for Wanda's European Skin Care Center. "Save your child a lifetime of waxing . . . and put the money in the bank for her college education instead!" The owner told the *New York Post* she'd seen two hundred child clients in 2007 and advised girls to begin waxing at six. You know, in the name of their future PhDs. Not only is this — needless to say — *not* even close to feminist, it's barbaric. A wax is, if nothing else, a choice a *woman* should make on her own, when she's at an appropriate age. And she should spend her formative years believing her body is perfect just the way nature gave it to her.

Yes, the waxing industry is an equal-opportunity torturer. That's why it's marketing more and more to men as well. Hairy chests are so *out* — see waxing scene in *The 40-Year-Old Virgin* for proof — and in some more metrosexual circles, that sentiment has moved farther south. We even have a fun term for it now: *man-scaping*. Those men who indulge in it do so for the same reason that women get bikini waxes — for their partners' benefit. So why sweat the feminism of it all if guys do it too? Like many issues of vanity, waxing, for men, can be more of a conscious choice, a nice extra something they do for their wives or girlfriends — not something they have to do just to compete with the male-run porn industry. For women, the norm in many parts of America, especially major metropolitan areas, is some pubic grooming, if not outright Brazilian waxing; to choose not to participate is the deviation. For most men, it's a far less fraught choice.

It should be noted, too, that more compulsive grooming for men is not necessarily good news for feminism. The movement, as we see it, means not only winning freedoms for women that are equal to men's but also claiming *more* freedom of expression for everyone, allowing both sexes to play with identity, gender, and appearance. Male models now have to wax their chests just like female models have always had to shave their legs and as they now must wax their bikini areas, but that doesn't mean feminism is winning. In fact, the shrinking range of acceptable appearances in advertising is a loss for feminism. Feminists fight for everyone's right to look how he or she wants to look, whether that's shaven, waxed, or hairy.

For now, women facing the decision to Brazilian wax or not to Brazilian wax must weigh their motives against their feminist principles. "If you wax, you pull [feminism] out by the roots, and therefore you're no longer a feminist and you have to turn in your Feminist Membership Card," one blogger wrote on Feministe.us (probably at least a little facetiously). A commenter, however, offered a solution: "We could go around in coveralls, with glasses on, with shaved heads and hairy legs. If we were the only females around, [men] would find us charming and devastating. We don't HAVE to cripple ourselves for their approval, or even wax our butt-holes."

It's a personal choice. Because a waxed bikini area is hardly a publicly displayed decision for most of us, it doesn't make the same kind of societal statement that a boob job, or even makeup or fashion, does. Done for the right reasons, waxing isn't a feminist issue at all, but a matter of preference. (Surely improving your own sexual stimulation is worth a few feminist points.) But done for the wrong reasons, it can quickly become antifeminist. Be sure your reasons are the right ones.

Questions to Consider Before You Wax

1. Why are you doing it? Is it because of pressure from your lover, your peers, or society? Or just because you prefer it

to not waxing? (Hint: We'd declare you clear for the landing strip only if you truly prefer to be waxed, whether it's because it improves your sex life, it simplifies your everyday shaving routine, or you just plain like it.)

2. Is it in your budget to spend sixty to a hundred dollars per month on this extra service? Can you maintain it?

3. Can you have a no-nonsense conversation with your waxer about how much of your hair you'd like to keep? Because if you can't bring yourself to talk about labia — even in coded terms like *undercarriage* and *front-to-back* — you aren't ready to go Brazilian.

4. Do you have an impeccable upscale salon or spa — as recommended by many, many friends and reputable publications — to which you can go for your wax? If not, *forget it*. Please. We beg you.

5. Does waxing make you want to vajazzle? If so, sorry, you've lost us, Jennifer Love Hewitt.

6. Does waxing make you want to get labial plastic surgery or re-hymenization? If so, sorry, we cannot support you on that either. Your vagina deserves more respect. Lines must be drawn.

7. Does your waxing regimen inspire you to take your eight-year-old in for a similar procedure? In the name of sisterhood, we *must* stop you there. Let her grow up and decide for herself.

8. Do you have a reasonable tolerance for pain? If you're super-sensitive, this might not be for you. That said, we'll also tell you that the first time is much worse than the subsequent

visits for maintenance if you stay on a regular monthly schedule. Any more frequent and there won't be enough hair to
pull; any less frequent and you're back to having enough
hair to make it really hurt.

Sexy Feminist Action Plan: Self-Help for Your Vagina

1. Visit a website like MyVag.net or VaginaVerite.com to explore all sorts of sex-positive, empowering ways to feel good
about your lady parts, waxed or not.

2. Watch some woman-friendly porn. Realize you don't have to
do any of what those women are doing if you don't want to,
but check out the variations in lady parts either way.
HotMoviesforHer.com and Dodsonandross.com, the website
of second-wave orgasm educator extraordinaire Betty Dodson, are good places to start.

3. Learn the lingo and research good salons if you do decide
to go.

4. Ask your lover what he or she likes about your vagina.
Straight men and gay women tend to like them more than
some straight women do and can help you love yourself a little more.

5. Talk to your lover about what he or she prefers, grooming-
wise, and why. This doesn't mean you have to do everything your lover asks for; it just means you're getting his or
her expectations out in the open so you don't find out at the
wrong time (like when you're watching porn with your boy-

friend and he says he wishes you looked more like the chick onscreen, in which case you may ask him to leave, with or without giving him a kick in the ball sack first) or find out the hard way (like when you undergo the pain of your first Brazilian as a surprise for your lover only to find out he *hates* waxing as much as you do). Also, feel free to tell him what goes into making your lady parts so smooth — go ahead, be dramatic about the eighty-dollar cost and every bit of the pain. He should know what you go through, and he should be just fine with seeing you between appointments. Then talk about what *you* prefer and why. This is your chance to tell him you'd love to go to certain places on him if he could, perhaps, take a trimmer to them. Or to tell him you love his hairy, Tom Selleck chest and hope he's never inspired to visit a salon after a late-night viewing of *The 40-Year-Old Virgin*.

6. Consider shaving if you like the idea of going bare but hate the idea of waxing or find it prohibitively expensive. For the record, both of the authors prefer waxing for its smooth and lasting effects, but a friend of ours has been Brazilian shaving for years and tells us: "I figured out how to do it by paying special attention to how they do the waxing. It's all about pulling your skin tight before you start shaving — much the same way they do when you get waxed. It takes a little practice, but I do it all the time very quickly with absolutely no issues. It's not as perfect as a Brazilian, but it saves me the pain, time, and money. So for me, it's well worth it."

7. Talk to your girlfriends about waxing. You'll find out what other women are doing and not doing, and you'll have much more fun than you would having your 732nd conversation about your annoying boss and your friend's noncommittal boyfriend.

THREE

PLASTIC SURGERY: CAN YOU?

I N MAY 2011, A YOUNG mother sat down for a TV interview to defend giving her eight-year-old daughter regular Botox injections. She said it was the edge her girl needed on the ultra-competitive beauty-pageant circuit. Those mussy lines on her face just wouldn't do. According to her mom, this eight-year-old's lips were too weak as well, so she added Restylane injections to the child's regular beauty routine, which also included spray tanning, teeth whitening, and virgin waxing — waxing the child's body (legs, arms, armpits, labia) to permanently prevent hair growth. (See chapter 2 for more on that.) In June of the same year, the mother of a seven-year-old embarked on her own media tour to defend a gift she'd recently given her daughter: an IOU for breast implants.

Weird plastic-surgery stories are nothing new. For decades, there have been tales of "cat women" so addicted to plastic surgery that they've erased the humanity from their features. But at least these are grown women making choices — choices that have feminist consequences, and we'll get to those in a bit. But little girls don't know that their faces have lines, that body hair is ugly, or that their breasts will be inadequate unless someone feeds them these messages. What have we done to women that their idea of beautiful is so twisted it causes them to subject their children to needles and scalpels? Alas, dads are doing it too. In a 2011 episode of the talk show *Anderson*, a male plastic surgeon defended giving his teenage daughter breast implants and a nose job. Sigh.

For starters, our culture presents plastic surgery as a symbol of the rich and famous, rather than as real surgery with serious consequences. We're assaulted by tabloid-cover headlines of "Plastic Surgery Horror Stories Revealed!" that make the results of botched surgeries punch lines rather than cautionary tales. Talk shows and even the evening news — once a place where one could actually get *news* — love to analyze a celebrity's new boobs, lifted butt, botched Botox job, or rumors of any of the above. Worst of all is reality television, which sometimes could be mistaken for advertising for surgical enhancements — see *The Real Housewives of* [Anywhere], *Keeping Up with the Kardashians*, and (horror of horrors) *Bridalplasty*. That last one pits brides-to-be against one another to compete in challenges that yield plastic-surgery procedures (winning?). The woman who receives the most procedures (now the "prettiest") is granted her dream wedding, courtesy of TV's seediest, most sexist pimp, the E! Network. We thought the worst of this kind of trash was over when *The Swan* was booed off television in 2005 for its horrific premise: carving insecure women to pieces and then making them compete in a beauty pageant.

This type of exploitative fare is likely to cause even marginal feminists to flinch. But plastic surgery is still one of our more polarizing debates. On the one hand, some argue that because feminism gives us the right to govern our bodies, women can indulge in cosmetic surgery and even feel empowered by it. Altering ourselves for ourselves, and no one else.

On the other hand, we have the argument that women wanting to change themselves are feeling pressured to do so because of the ever-present sexist beauty ideal shoved down their throats — perfect women in magazines, movies, television shows, and, of course, porn (here's yet another example of how porn makes women judge themselves). By undergoing elective surgery — or filling up on injectables — women are mangling the message feminists have worked so hard to spread. We don't need your corsets, your miracle cures for aging, your diets, or your knives — women are strong, beautiful, and powerful just as they are.

Can a woman believe these things about herself — and other women — and still consider plastic surgery? How do we reconcile even a small aesthetic tweak — laser resurfacing; maybe just one round of Botox (just one!) — with feminist principles that reject the need for such improvements? And is getting a few Botox shots less of a feminist betrayal than getting breast implants? The feminist dilemma here is this: Is a woman's right to pursue a positive body image worth the cost of getting there?

LIFESAVER VERSUS BOOB BOOSTER

Cosmetic surgery has been a part of our culture for a long time, but it hasn't always been so controversial — or so gruesome. As early as 800 B.C., doctors were performing cosmetic procedures. Skin grafts were recorded in India more than four thousand years ago. Wars and their disfiguring effects motivated advances in plastic surgery. Soldiers returning home from the bloody battles were given the chance to have their former selves reconstructed. Plastic surgery has been a miracle for children with cleft palates, and for accident and burn victims. This is where cosmetic surgery is an art form — and sometimes saves lives. And in the cases of mastectomy patients, individuals born with genetic abnormalities that affect life functioning, or those who feel they were born the wrong gender, plastic surgery can help them inhabit their basic identities and can end devastating, lifelong psychological struggles. When making a physical cosmetic change is necessary to find or recover one's sense of self, it's an act of personal human rights.

These cases are a small percentage of the plastic surgeries performed every year, however. Elective cosmetic procedures — those to enhance breasts, shave noses, erase wrinkles, suck fat, and re-shape women's vaginas — are the bread and butter of this $10 billion industry.

Breast implants in particular are central to the feminist-or-not debate over plastic surgery. Our society is boob obsessed, and it seems some women will do anything to make their breasts look like the perfect, perky D-cups shoved in their faces everywhere they turn. Breasts are the sexual characteristics that publicly define womanhood, so this obsession makes sense, even if it's unhealthy. When a woman's breasts change due to dramatic weight gain or loss, pregnancy, or surgery, many argue that the woman herself changes too, and she might want some surgical help in dealing with that. "Let's face it: breasts — their shape, size, and sensation — play an integral role in how women define themselves as women," says Dr. Haideh Hirmand, a plastic surgeon who specializes in breast surgery, the most common cosmetic surgical procedure in the United States. "Many women whose breasts have significantly changed express a consistent theme of having lost an integral part of their physique that made them feel whole as a woman. They didn't know it until it was lost."

Of course, many other women (the majority, we hope) don't feel lost or incomplete no matter what changes their breasts go through. A friend of ours who has maintained her solid sense of self while living in Los Angeles (fake-boob central) and working in the spa and beauty industry says it perfectly: "As an undeniably small-breasted woman who has seen plenty of changes due to two pregnancies and years of breastfeeding, I've never even entertained the idea of getting implants. Would it be nice to have bigger boobs? Sure. Do I feel like the size of my breasts defines me as a woman? No way."

Hirmand argues that her patients are on a quest to restore their vitality, but where do we draw the line when it comes to supporting surgery as an offshoot of feminism? The problem lies in that desire to alter. Medical and extreme psychological necessity aside, a woman who has cosmetic surgery wants to change her appearance to resemble someone else — be it a favorite celebrity or a younger version of herself. This desire wasn't inborn. Media-influenced brainwashing tells women they have to look a certain way. Stopping that message is the collective feminist mission.

BRAINWASHED TO BEAUTIFY: HOW SEXIST CULTURE MAKES WOMEN GO UNDER THE KNIFE

This message that women are flawed and must improve their looks (to attract men, natch) is fed to them at earlier and earlier ages. Children want their hair — and makeup — to look like their dolls', which resemble disproportionate grown women. Teenage girls want breast implants instead of cars for their sixteenth birthdays. In 2010, nearly 220,000 plastic-surgery procedures were performed on females eighteen and younger. Women in their twenties are already signed up for the endless cycle of Botox treatments. And women as young as thirty are going under the knife to "turn back the clock," an expression that is as disgusting as it is enraging — not to mention that it's in defiance of basic physics. It's a catchy phrase used to advertise everything from eye cream to vitamins, and it supports an impossible standard at best and an infantilized sexual ideal at worst. Younger is sexier, duh.

Young and sexy today also likely means "broke." It's no secret women are the target market for all things cosmetic, and this ever-more-extreme expense can bleed them dry, especially when they're making only 70 percent of what men make as it is. Women spend tens of billions of dollars to beautify themselves, and that's not even including the cost of new pairs of jeans. So how can women afford this? Um, we can't. More than half of female plastic-surgery patients have incomes below $25,000 a year. So while men spend their extra money on new cars, real estate, and maybe savings for the future — plus plenty of other superficial and silly things, to be sure — women making less than minimum wage are leveraging their tiny net worths on carving "better" versions of themselves. This is hardly advancing women's collective wealth and power.

Extreme cosmetic procedures also happen to be a serious threat to health. To understand why plastic surgery is a feminist issue, we need to look at what it is — the ugly, bloody details. Imagery surrounding plastic surgery more often than not focuses on the "after." Women showcasing smooth, tight new parts are shown smiling and dancing, usually on a beach. The reality of what they must endure to achieve the end result of smoother, tighter, younger (and happier?) are details usually confined to the doctor's office. Here's what the most popular procedures entail:

RHINOPLASTY

What it is: The good old-fashioned nose job is now so common, it's often used as a comedic aside in film, TV, and standup acts — and the butt of the joke is always a woman. Remember poor Jennifer Grey's ribbing and effective ousting from the entertainment industry after she got the nose her agents and managers no doubt talked her into? Here's what they're laughing at: After the patient is sedated, her nose is cut free from the cartilage so doctors can get to work sawing and hammering it into a new shape. Advertised recovery time is a few weeks, but most cases require six months to a year, and often a follow-up procedure is necessary to fix any imper-

Check Out Receipt

Victorville City Library
760-245-4222
http://ci.victorville.ca.us/library

Thursday, May 24, 2018 5:15:23 PM
Elizalde-Garcia, Jessica

Item: 81483000658832
Title: How successful people grow : 15 way
s to get ahead in life
Call no.: 158 MAX 2014
Material: Book
Due: 06/14/2018

Item: 81483000465041
Title: Sexy feminism : a girl's guide to l
ove, success, and style
Call no.: 305.42 ARM 2013
Material: Book
Due: 06/14/2018

Total items: 2

Thank You!

72

fections or complications — including infections, blockages, and trouble breathing.

Feminist analysis: There are medical indications for rhinoplasty, such as a deviated septum that causes breathing problems or a deformity caused by trauma to the area. In these cases, yes, get your nose fixed so it can function. But if you want a nose job so you can look more like someone else or less like yourself, we'd like for you to instead find a way to fall in love with the girl in the mirror — because she's kind of awesome just as she is. She's at least as awesome as Barbra Streisand or Sarah Jessica Parker, beautiful women and feminist icons who scoffed at public pressure to go under the knife.

BREAST AUGMENTATION

What it is: Somewhere between 1950s cone-shaped bras and *Playboy*, the American model of a perfect woman grew into bra size 32-DD. Roughly 1 percent of women in the United States achieve this naturally. Anyone in the other 99 percent who wishes to get these popular fun bags must go under general anesthesia and have a surgeon insert the implants through an incision made under the breast, in the armpit, around the nipple, or through the navel. While surgical techniques for breast augmentation have advanced, resulting in minimal scarring and faster recovery time, there is still a "definite certainty of implant failure," says the website of plastic surgeon Richard V. Dowden. So that means a guaranteed second, third, or even fourth surgery, depending on how long you keep your implants. And if you're going to wind up taking them out —

requiring another surgery and additional enhancements to fix sagging and scarring — what's the point?

Feminist analysis: The invention of artificial breasts is a miracle for women whose natural ones are damaged or removed due to illness or injury. And breast surgery is an integral step in gender reassignment for those desperately trying to be their authentic selves. But the average breast-augmentation recipient is a typical-sized woman who just thought she needed to look better. Finding a way to feel comfortable with our own breasts — no matter their size and shape — is something we all need to work on if we're ever going to banish this absurd (and impossible) figure ideal. To start you off, we have a pep talk for your boobs:

Small cups: Girls, you don't know how good you've got it. Yes, the world bombards you with images of breasts three times larger than yours, but come on: that's not you. You are low maintenance, forever perky, and lucky enough to never have to deal with underwire. Rooney Mara, Gwyneth Paltrow, and Zoë Saldana are your heroines. And these are some of the sexiest women alive — women who can wear necklines as low as they want without a care in the world.

Medium cups: The B-cup is the most common naturally occurring size in the world, so there's a predetermined reason you are the size and shape you are. No, being just a little bigger will not make you perfect; you're already there. Jessica Biel, Beyoncé, and Sarah Jessica Parker (her own nose *and* boobs!) are natural goddesses.

Large cups: We know, it can suck to be ogled — ugh! But your size serves a purpose: your breasts are likely proportionate to the rest of your curves — you were born to be curvy, a reason to celebrate. Don't be ashamed of yourself because everyone pays a little too much attention to you. Embrace it. Wear fitted sweaters because you feel good in them. Jennifer Hudson, Queen Latifah, and Christina Hendricks are your well-endowed sisters.

Now, we understand there's a difference between being well-endowed and having problematically large breasts. Many women have breasts so large that they cause back and neck problems, and that's in addition to the psychological damage caused by constant attention and criticism (typically beginning at a young age). Same goes for the small percentage of women with virtually no breasts at all. (And we mean really, truly nonexistent for hormonal reasons.) For these women, breast surgery can improve their physical and mental health. (Queen Latifah, in fact, underwent a breast reduction to change her F-cup breasts to DD-cups. She's still voluptuous and fabulous.) We're all for that. There's an extreme point at which most medical procedures make sense; that's the kind of extreme point we're talking about here.

LIPOSUCTION

What it is: After general anesthesia is administered, a doctor makes incisions in the skin, then vacuums fat from the desired areas. Liposuction has one of the highest mortality rates of any cosmetic procedure, due to complications associated with anesthesia (for example, a blood clot in the lung) and patients' desire to have too much liposuction done at once. Multiple liposuctions — especially coupled with additional cosmetic-surgery procedures — can put undue stress on the heart and lead to cardiac arrest.

Feminist analysis: We're not going to say we love cellulite. But we are learning to accept it. Nearly every woman has it — it's just the genetic card we're dealt with that second X-chromosome (though men get cellulite too). We'd love to make it and excess fat magically disappear, but here's the thing: Fat and cellulite come back. There is no such thing as a permanent quick fix to this biological reality. Subjecting yourself to torture akin to a vignette in the latest *Saw* film to lose a few inches is not an empowering experience. It's torture porn and this is your real life.

TUMMY TUCK

What it is: Make no mistake: this procedure is intense. It involves an incision from hipbone to hipbone, after which the skin is peeled back, the fat is sucked out, your bellybutton is cut out and saved for the new location the surgeon will make for it, the extra skin is cut off, the remainder is stretched into place like a new drumhead, the bellybutton is repositioned, and you're stitched back together. Patients must walk hunched over for several weeks before the skin loosens enough for them to stand upright. Recovery time for this procedure is longer than for most — six months in the best cases. And even though for the first few weeks you're practically unable to move, you'd better move, or you could get a blood clot that has a 30 percent chance of killing you.

Feminist analysis: Forget the gruesome visual of being sliced in half then put back together again. This procedure has been dubbed the mommy tuck, as pressure has mounted for new mothers to snap back into their pre-baby bodies (you know, like the fa-

mous, rich celebrities, with their teams of personal trainers, dieti-
cians, and nannies, do). The rate of tummy tucks has risen more
than 80 percent since 2000, and almost half are performed on
women in their twenties and thirties. Internet message boards and
forums have dubbed the mommy tuck a must-do procedure after
a woman has a kid, as if it were on the new-parent checklist along
with babyproofing the house and starting a college fund. Reality
check: pregnancy and childbirth change your body — and thank
goodness for that! You can't achieve making — and delivering — a
new human being without significant physical changes. Granted,
some women are left with more changes than others, but submit-
ting to an operation that leaves you essentially crippled doesn't
seem like the best idea for a mother caring for a new baby. Considering that one of feminism's founding principles is that women
should be allowed to choose if and when they want to be mothers,
we owe it to ourselves and the movement to understand what becoming a mother involves — stretch marks and all. Personal note
from one feminist mother: stretch marks and a little loose skin are
a pretty reasonable tradeoff for an amazing new person who will
change your life forever.

LABIAPLASTY (AKA DESIGNER VAGINAS)

What it is: Labiaplasty — which entails cutting or reshaping the
labia minora or labia majora to the desired tightness — is now on
the menu of services in most plastic surgeons' offices.

Feminist analysis: Thanks a lot, porn — yeah, again. It's not bad
enough that women are seeking out the EE-cup breast implants

of porn stars, now they want porn vaginas, which have most assuredly been altered with makeup, film-editing techniques, and the like. Yes, there are cases in which a woman's labia are disfiguringly long, causing pain or sexual dysfunction. This is a health condition that can be corrected with surgery, at the woman's discretion. Wanting your vagina to resemble Jenna Jameson's isn't cause for cutting. Consider whom these nips and tucks are for. Are *you* the one who wants the "re-virginization" treatment (an add-on that requires suturing together the remnants of the hymen so a woman can have the bloody, painful experience of losing her virginity all over again)? Really? If a man isn't happy with the vagina you've given him access to, he can take his business elsewhere. You and your beautiful-just-as-it-is vagina can do better. Remember that people in other parts of the world are risking their lives to save girls and women from forced genital mutilation. We owe it to them as much as to ourselves to respect our bodies.

BOTOX AND INJECTABLES

What it is: Needles insert the desired agent — botulin to paralyze facial muscles or synthetic fillers to plump lips or cheeks.

Feminist analysis: We've been used to needles since childhood immunizations. Is this that big a deal? Yes. Even though injections are among the least invasive procedures, they're high on our feminist watch list. Consider the motivation for any woman to fill her face — her face! — with poison or synthetic material to distort it from any semblance of normal. There are no medical exceptions here or humanitarian cases. These procedures are purely cosmetic and the motivation the same: make me look younger. This is not the message we should be sending women and young girls. Plus, a 2010 USC/Duke University medical study revealed that getting Botox may actually take away a woman's ability to feel emotions. By restricting facial expressions, you lose the natural, youthful exuberance that actually makes you *feel* younger. Not to mention that Botox face, past a certain point, doesn't make a woman look "younger" so much as "of a different species."

So, yes, feminism has given us the right to govern our own bodies and take pride in our appearance. But hacking and chopping ourselves to get there is hardly something to brag about; in fact, it makes our heads (and hearts) hurt. To advocate for women to love, cherish, and respect themselves — including the package they came in — we stand on the side of no scalpels or needles unless there's a medical or truly deep, otherwise unsolvable psychological need. Understanding why women are brainwashed to want to look like pretend-perfect twenty-somethings and doing away with that mindset is the call to action we need to answer.

Besides, putting plastic surgeons out of the cosmetic-procedure business is our best defense, as a gender, against this industry's constant assault on our bodies and psyches. There's nothing more feminist than that.

Sexy Feminist Action Plan: Invest in Yourself, Not New Boobs

We know it's a long road for women to reach a collective self-confidence that makes plastic surgery a rarity. Here are a few guidelines to help you along on your journey.

1. **Stop watching salacious reality television.** We know; it's addictive. But while you think you're watching to indulge in a little schadenfreude, your subconscious is absorbing the message these shows send: women are most valuable as beautiful, perfectly proportioned, super-sexual dummies crafted and carved to serve as men's playthings. Your mind deserves better than this.

2. **Make happiness a priority.** Yes, this sounds like a schmaltzy fortune-cookie scrawl, but the truth is that we don't take enough time for ourselves in our busy lives. This relates to our feelings of insecurity and desire to please. If we are happier with ourselves, we won't be looking to plastic surgeons to give us a miracle. When you look in the mirror and see something you don't like, most of the time it's the inside that needs help, not the outside. Find a way to work on that inner smile. Take up yoga; learn to meditate; or spend extra time talking to a true, trusted friend about your feelings.

3. **Investigate natural alternatives to plastic surgery.** Look, we're all for searching for the eye cream that banishes crow's-feet or the workout that feels great and still burns fat. We're human and we want to improve ourselves. But rather than looking to invasive measures, consider acupuncture, a healthy and rigorous workout regimen, or natural skin care that works. Or even get a haircut. It's hard not to feel fabulous with a new do — and getting bangs is way less invasive than getting Botox.

4. **Don't be afraid of therapy.** If you find yourself overwhelmed with feelings of self-loathing or can't look in the mirror without imagining what some cosmetic enhancements would do,

consult a therapist to help you understand the motivations behind your desires. Cosmetic surgery isn't like an eyebrow piercing you can let close up later. Pieces of your body are removed, never to return. These are pretty damn permanent procedures; it's worth a little mental-health investment first.

5. **Do your due diligence.** If you're going to go under the knife — for one of the feminist-approved reasons cited above — you owe it to yourself to know what you're getting. And please be certain you really, truly want this.

   - Talk to a therapist — get a clean bill of mental health before you go in.

   - Look at the photos — even the grossest ones. Investigate procedural images and videos of what you intend to have done. You need to understand what can go wrong and realize you may have to live with that.

   - Find a good doctor — don't even think about going to Craigslist or calling an 800 number from an ad you saw in your alt weekly. Look up doctors online, review their credentials and patient testimonials, and make sure their certifications are up to date. Any doctor worth seeing will have this information available.

   - Ask yourself — yes, again — do I really want this? Does your flat chest cause you mental anguish or are you proportionally petite? Does your deviated septum interfere with your breathing or do you just want to be rid of the small bump on your nose?

6. **Use your favorite asset to give the rest of you a pep talk.** So you bemoan your small breasts or can't stand the fullness in your hips. We can't give you a magic pill to make

those ingrained insecurities disappear. But we bet there's a feature of yours you love — and love showing off. Don't be modest; the truth is evident in your addiction to low-rise jeans (your abs and lower back are killer!), your collection of one-shouldered tops (your clavicle is a thing of sculptural beauty!), your short skirts (your legs stop traffic), your open-toed shoes (you've been told more than once how sexy your feet are), or your wrap dresses (people make that double-handed swerve-y gesture to describe your natural hourglass). You give these assets plenty of love because you know they work for you — and you know how to work them. Lend the rest of your body some of that positive energy every now and then. Know we were all given the proportions that are right for us. This means most of us aren't meant to have a perfect ass, a flat stomach, *and* a big chest all at once. The models who do are either genetic freaks or plastic-surgery victims. Deal.

Feminist Confessions: What I Learned from a Laser Facial Peel

I spent years with a laser facial treatment on my wish list, but it remained far from possible for most of my twenties and thirties, thanks to the prohibitive $2,000 cost. But when I got my first book deal while I was still working at a well-paying full-time job, I found myself flush with disposable income. Regular taxis, luxurious dinners out, and overpriced designer jeans became part of my new reality, and I decided I would also choose one big-ticket indulgence before socking the rest of my newfound money away in my savings account. The winner was a laser treatment to smooth away the evidence of hard-fought battles with terrible teen acne.

I have a fancy dermatologist, the kind who's quoted regularly in women's magazines and who's worth the hour-plus trip on the subway from Brooklyn to the Upper East Side of Manhattan, so I wasn't worried about safety. The nurse who handles the outpatient cosmetic procedures at the office told me to expect some discomfort. She also advised me to take a few days to a week off work for recovery, because my face would be a little red, "like a sunburn" — a mantra everyone in the office would repeat often throughout the process. I've had sunburn. I could live with that.

But I am here to tell you that in cosmetic-surgery land, all reality is distorted — not just the shape of your breasts or the texture of your skin, but the basic agreed-upon-by-all-of-society definitions of words and perceptions of what is reasonable. A few lessons I learned from undergoing even the most minor of cosmetic procedures:

1. ***Discomfort* means "searing pain."** I had imagined, with all this talk of discomfort and sunburns, that this thing would be like having someone point, like, one of those laser pens you use in presentations at my face until it stung a little, and then I'd be sent home. It turns out the doctor was actually *burning my face off* so the skin could grow back slightly smoother.

2. ***A few days to a week off* means "at least a week."** I had scheduled myself to go back to work five days after my procedure, which meant I'd taken three days plus a weekend. I was lucky enough to have a job at a magazine where I could hide in my office under the guise of

writing, but I wonder what any of my poor coworkers who caught a glimpse of me must have thought about the chunks of skin still in the process of molting off my face at the time.

3. **They are not kidding when they advise you to have someone take you home afterward.** I thought, *For a sunburn? Surely that can withstand my taking a taxi ride home without assistance.* Then I found myself with my face wrapped in gauze like a mummy, oozing everywhere under the June sun, hailing a cab near Central Park. I'm glad I didn't invite my new boyfriend to witness this event, but I did wish I'd dragged a friend along with me.

4. **"May require multiple treatments for desired results"? No, thanks.** My dermatologist wants to do it one more time to achieve the perfect results promised on the brochure — in fact, this is included in my original price, so I'd be getting my money's worth — but I can't bring myself to do it. It was just too painful for the results, and I've found one of those nice spot-erasing creams that works enough to make me happy. Going through this whole thing made me come to terms with my face as it is — there are still a few marks here and there, but now that I know what it takes to get rid of them, I don't mind them as much.

— *Jennifer Keishin Armstrong*

FOUR

VANITY IS NOT A FEMINIST SIN

THERE ARE OBVIOUS conflicts between feminism and the American beauty ideal. It's become such a powerful force that women are hardly ever seen in public sans makeup — and they're certainly never presented without it in media and entertainment. This expectation that females always must be made up contributes to low self-esteem in most of us and further excludes the portion of the population that doesn't look like what magazines and movies proclaim is beautiful (that would be most of us again). It's a pressure that has been weighing on women for decades.

"The beauty myth, like many ideologies of femininity, mutates to meet new circumstances and checkmates women's attempts to increase their power," writes Naomi Wolf in an introduction to the 2002 update of *The Beauty Myth*, published ten years after the original. Another decade later, we're still mutating. Porn now influences all of our aesthetic choices and has made huge breasts, platinum hair, and hairless vaginas seem standard, which means many women not naturally endowed with those features are altering themselves to fit the new-and-improved model. These are things worth feminist uprising.

But don't throw out your Sephora rewards card just yet. We can find feminist merit in beauty products by looking at their origins. In doing so, we discover makeup being used as power, and female pioneers creating one of the most profitable industries in the world.

Makeup hardly began as a way to mark women as the prettier sex — that's a modern Western phenomenon. It was far more practical than that. The first people to use makeup were the Egyptians, but it wasn't thanks to Cleopatra. Long before Cleo, men and women slathered on moisturizer and smudged kohl around their orbital bones to protect themselves from the desert's sun, wind, and insects. But like many cultural practices with utilitarian origins, applying makeup eventually became a trend, and one with status. The wealthiest Egyptians (again, both men and women) lined their eyes in black, painted their lids in brilliant green shadows made from minerals, stained their cheeks and lips, and kept scented oils in jeweled bottles. You could tell the wealth of a person by the makeup tools with which he or she was buried.

Similarly, China's earliest form of makeup — nail polish made from beeswax, gelatin, and egg — was used as a way to distinguish among classes, not between genders. Fast-forward a few centuries, and Europeans were also using makeup as a class identifier, but gender segregation began to creep in. It was Queen Elizabeth I who popularized face powder to achieve the then ideal of beauty: pale and delicate — the lighter the skin, the higher the social rank. Up until the nineteenth century, women were powdering with a toxic cocktail containing lead. But that's not half as bad as the technique that fashionable sixth-century women used to appear beautifully (to them) pale: bleeding themselves.

Not everyone celebrated these adornment trends. Queen Elizabeth's female followers often had to hide their "painting," as it was known, from men, who found the practice sinful. In the Middle Ages, religious leaders decreed makeup blasphemous. They ostracized the women who used it, calling them whores — and often treating them like it. This was, of course, a general problem with the Middle Ages. During the Victorian era, the popularity of cosmetics diminished. Women who wore makeup were assumed to be of low moral standards. Cosmetics were viewed as "the devil's making."

At the turn of the century, women declared their independence from men by expressing themselves creatively, often through makeup. Publishing also began to wield some influence. The earliest magazines and journals were already instructing women how to properly exercise, diet, and use hair and makeup products to be beautiful.

Beginning around World War I, women started exercising their buying power and asserted their independence by purchasing makeup, hair products, and trendy clothing. In 1920s America, women wore false eyelashes and red lips along with flapper garb to celebrate their freedom. In the 1940s, though, the U.S. government issued a bill banning most makeup items and reforming the production and packaging of the rest. Now American women were urged to support the men-at-arms by limiting their cosmetics consumption. These ladies weren't having it. The demand from women forced the cosmetics industry to reinvent itself and reformulate beauty products made from Uncle Sam–approved ingredients and packaging. Glamour lived on! Rosie could be the riveter, but she wasn't giving up her lipstick.

Before the second-wave feminist revolution, women used makeup as a way to control their appearance, since little else was in their control. The 1950s and 1960s brought big drama in makeup trends — sultry eyes, bold lips, and hair in volumes it had never risen to before. Women may have been relegated to being stay-at-home mothers and housewives, but they were embracing their beauty freedoms. The beauty business also allowed a woman to earn a living and establish independence. Mary Kay and Avon gave women the opportunity to be entrepreneurs and thrive in a society that had made June Cleaver the epitome of what a female *should* be. Were these businesses so successful because makeup and beauty products were considered elements of the domestic realm, which meant men didn't pay them much mind? Perhaps. But who cares? These industrious women were creating new wealth for themselves in a way that had previously been inaccessible to them. It set the precedent for an industry that would employ millions of women.

It wasn't until the 1970s and the height of the second-wave feminist movement that women started rejecting makeup as being part of the system set up to keep them down. (Though this was the same decade in which makeup was first made for women of different skin tones, which was a kind of small civil rights victory.) Protesting the beauty business — and its billions of products women had grown to love or at least had been lured into loving by omnipresent advertising — was an important part of feminist progress at this time. Feminists rallied most against the images projected through the industry's ads. A woman had to look like either Marilyn Monroe or a rail-thin runway model to be considered beautiful. Or, more to the point, a woman who didn't look like either ideal might as well not exist, as these were the only images shown in advertising for products ranging from hair remover to shampoo. The idea was to make regular women feel inadequate so they'd run out and buy the advertised products in hopes of getting a little closer to looking like a movie star.

About this same time, Hugh Hefner made *Playboy* not just a hit at the newsstands but a lifestyle brand that men and women alike were swallowing whole. While *Playboy*'s advocacy for female sexual liberation is something we can get behind, its continued depiction of women as sexual playthings for men is not, nor is Hefner's overdone (and enduring) preferred female aesthetic. *Playboy* used women (most of them Barbie-like) as pretty little objects to entertain and please men. *The Beauty Myth* was inspired by this sexist message — and by the way the world fell for it. Author Naomi Wolf called out magazines, advertisers, and women themselves for putting up with an artificial ideal no woman could achieve.

Feminists had to reject the products that promoted this image or no one would have noticed the harm being done. So some of them threw out their makeup, stopped shaving their legs, and refused to wear restrictive, patriarchal items such as high heels and bras as a way to combat this forced picture of perfection. For the record: Feminists protesting the 1968 Miss America pageant threw many items of patriarchal oppression — girdles, cosmetics, high heels, and bras — into a "freedom" trash can, but they never lit a match. A photo of a woman hurling a bra into the can coupled with a flippant inaccurate caption created the bra-burning stereotype that still thrives today. In any case, it was protests such as this that were needed to make the world hear the message: Being a woman and feeling beautiful is about more than eyeliner and cleavage.

The next generation of feminists got it — Wolf's screed against packaged beauty is among the works credited for kicking off what would become known as feminism's third wave — but they brought back the makeup too. One of the third wave's defining features was the large number of lipstick feminists whose major agenda item was debunking the image of the sexless feminist by embracing fashion and makeup. These days, we don't see it as an either-or issue; women can choose to indulge in products or they can go without, their feminism intact. Do your real feminist work in painted face or plain while remaining ever watchful of the images the cosmetics industry feeds you.

So, yes, you *can* be a feminist and love mascara, rock red lips, or always smell of a signature scent. These are feminist acts if the image you're projecting reflects the individual on the inside, rather than an externally imposed one no woman could achieve. Feminist teacher and blogger Erin Z. puts it nicely: "I love makeup! And I use it as an important power tool in what I like to think of as my gender performativity."

MAKING OVER FEMINISM: BEAUTY'S PLACE IN THE MOVEMENT

Expression through makeup can be exhilarating. "One of the things that defines us as women in a positive way is we get to enjoy the colorful aesthetic — and the fun — of beauty," says Vivian Diller, PhD, a clinical psychologist and author of *Face It: What Women* Really *Feel as Their Looks Change and What to Do About It.*

The millions of products on the market today mask imperfections, smell delicious, make us sparkle, and on top of that, they're literally playthings — eye-shadow palettes in gorgeous cases with rhinestones; lip-gloss samplers in a rainbow of shades and flavors; bronzers with retractable brushes; nail polish in hologram hues . . . These items have become our favorite accessories, and with them we can paint our own identities and assert our uniqueness. They allow us to express our internal selves to the world just the way we want to or change the way people see us with the stroke of an eyeliner pencil. Just ask trans women, many of whom have mastered this easy, accessible method of self-expression.

Buying makeup can also be a feminist act if you support the right businesses. It's one of the few industries largely populated by female entrepreneurs. Most businesses that became beauty powerhouses were founded in the kitchens of women and turned into international corporations. Estée Lauder, Mary Kay, Avon, Helena Rubinstein, Elizabeth Arden, and Madame C. J. Walker still dominate the $10-billion-a-year industry nearly a century after the companies were founded. Though men now run many of these corporations — still, sadly, how business goes — women are often the pioneers, and the revolutionaries. Just a few of them:

- In 1968, magazine editor Carol Phillips consulted with Park Avenue dermatologist Dr. Norman Orentreich for a *Vogue* article entitled "Can Great Skin Be Created?" The article caught the attention of Estée Lauder, and Phillips was brought on board to help create the first dermatologist-developed skin-care line: Clinique.

- Bobbi Brown founded her makeup and skin-care line in 1991 on an aesthetic that's pretty darn feminist: enhancing — never masking — a woman's natural features. Her muted, skin-tone-based cosmetics and bestselling books and web tutorials taught millions of women how to apply makeup correctly (trust us, we weren't doing it right before) and master the art of "less is more." She was also one of the first to use African American models regularly in makeup ads and show them as brides, a practice until then unheard of even in the late twentieth century.

- Leslie Blodgett became CEO of a small company called Bare Escentuals in 1994. (It didn't hit QVC and every woman's makeup bag till the late 1990s.) The mineral-based line that addresses problem skin made headlines: Blodgett was committed to having real women represent the brand, and she hit the road to recruit American women throughout the United States. The ads featuring average Janes across the country helped create trust and loyalty for the brand.

- Maureen Kelly was a mom who wanted better makeup — chemical-free, easy to use, and cool-looking — when she

founded Tarte Cosmetics in 1999. It's now one of the fast-
est-growing brands in the business and donates part of its
proceeds to charity.

Still, the dilemma facing second-wave feminists is alive and well.
One must look at only a few ads in magazines to see why: A spring
color palette of eye shadow is being sold by a model with her
mouth agape and sex-hazed eyes. Every cream and lotion now has
the word *antiaging* on it (because God forbid we let nature take its
natural course), and all the ads feature teenage models showcasing the results! Pseudoscientific approaches are used to sell us on
a slew of face creams; some list ingredients such as so-called stem
cells — except that a look at the fine print tells you those are relatively useless cells from the stems of plants, not some kind of foun-
tain-of-youth miracle on par with the tissue-generating potential of
human embryonic stem cells. (Not that we'd like those in our face
creams either.) And who knows how they sold perfume before un-
derweight naked models were the norm?

Women are being told through these ads that being beautiful — and this specific version of beautiful — is the only way to
achieve happiness. Helena Rubinstein once said, "There are no
ugly women, only lazy ones." While this sounds like a motivational
speech, it's insulting. Women who choose not to spend any time at
all — much less hours — slathering on creams, concealers, and colors to look more like a Maybelline ad are ostracized for not fitting
into society and possibly even subjected to discrimination at work.
A 2011 study proclaimed that "makeup had significant positive effects on ratings of female facial attractiveness" and that "ratings of
competence increased significantly" for women who wore makeup
in the workplace. It must be noted that this study was funded by

Feminist Beauty Companies

Consider these feminist-minded companies the next time you need to stock up on your favorite products.

PeaceKeeper Cause-Metics: Founded on the principles of nonviolence and truthfulness, this company gives all of its after-tax distributable profits to charities that support women's health and human rights. It sells only products that come from companies that practice fair labor policies and do not test on animals: **Iamapeacekeeper.com**.

MAC: A favorite of stage actors and drag queens, MAC launched its line of VIVA Glam lipsticks and lip glosses in 1994 to contribute to HIV/AIDS research and treatment. The MAC AIDS Fund has raised more than $250 million worldwide through sales of VIVA Glam products, which are endorsed by sexy feminists Christina Aguilera, Cyndi Lauper, Mary J. Blige, and Lady Gaga. The lipsticks are freaking gorgeous and they last longer than most. So splurge — and save lives: **Maccosmetics.com**.

The Body Shop: Long gone are the days of the Body Shop's selling only hemp oils and patchouli perfumes (though you can still get those here too). This chain now has a complete modern line of face, body, and beauty products — from mango body butter to mineral makeup — all derived from natural ingredients and sourced from communities around the world to help sustain them. The company also has active campaigns to stop sex trafficking and domestic violence and to raise awareness of global HIV/AIDS: **Thebodyshop-usa.com**.

Procter & Gamble, which owns about half the world's beauty companies. But the message went viral anyway, appearing in women's magazines, beauty blogs, and news websites. When makeup and skin care are marketed as necessary, rather than optional, it takes away our freedom of choice.

Another problem with the beauty ideal sold through advertising is that it's a pale one. Products that promise a perfect skin tone might as well call it a *lighter* skin tone. Makeup ads may have their coffee-to-albino color spectrum on display in a tiny grid at the bottom of the page, but more often than not it's a white model selling the stuff above it.

TOXIC BEAUTY: DON'T DIE FOR
VANITY — OR EVEN GET A RASH

Even more troubling than how beauty products are sold is *what's* being sold. When's the last time you looked at the ingredients list of your mascara or shampoo? It's long, isn't it? The sad truth is most makeup is poison. Less than 20 percent of ingredients in cosmetics have even been assessed for safety, and terms such as *natural, organic,* and *herbal* are meaningless because the Food and Drug Administration does not regulate their use. This isn't some sexist conspiracy to take out the female of the species, but nonetheless it is plenty messed up. Why is it that food and pharmaceuticals are regulated but grooming products — even those made for babies — are not? The government isn't going to help us here, so it's our responsibility to know what we're putting on our skin (and thereby into our bodies) and to lobby against companies that make their money by hawking snake oils or poison. Check your brands on safecosmetics.org to make sure you know what you're buying. Even those brands whose missions and messages have feminist merit (including most of those we celebrate above) have a *lot* of work to do before they can be considered as kind to women's skin as they are to their souls. The best way to get what you want out of your products is to demand something better.

Extreme Makeup: What You Should Know

Lip plumpers: To give you that bee-sting pout, these products irritate your skin with corrosive chemicals. That tingling is your immune system coming to your defense by swelling the affected area. It's kind of like getting yourself punched in the face so you can have that smoky-eye look.

Permanent makeup: It's what it sounds like — a tiny needle injects dye under the skin of your eyes, lips, and — sometimes — your unmentionables (women have opted for permanent makeup on their labia to make them, you know, "pinker" — don't *even* get us started). If you're having remorse about that butterfly tattoo above your hip (so cool then, so tramp-stamp now), think how you'll feel about permanent lip liner or eyeliner in ten years.

Cellulite creams: Years of research on these products have proven over and over and over that they do . . . nothing (again, they're not regulated). Invest in a good pair of running shoes and get out on a trail instead. PS: Everyone has cellulite. Everyone. It's worth coming to terms with it.

Retinols: Otherwise known as vitamin A, the topical form of this wonder ingredient can erase wrinkles, freckles, and age spots through natural exfoliation (we are fans!). But for the love, get a prescription from a dermatologist. The over-the-counter products aren't concentrated enough to do much good, and a doctor will know which concentration is best for your skin.

Sexy Feminist Action Plan: Primp with Purpose

Saving the world one mascara tube at a time means buying, wearing, and researching your beauty consumption responsibly.

1. **Understand the feminist history of the beauty industry.** We can wear as much or as little makeup as we want today without fear of feminist failure because of the protests, boycotts, and bold statements of our second-wave sisters. They helped expose the beauty myth and raised awareness about the sometimes evil cosmetics industry. Appreciating the work that led to our freedom of expression makes each mascara stroke matter a little bit more.

2. **Carry on the feminist fight.** Don't accept subpar products that hurt your skin or your conscience. Know where your beauty essentials come from — research companies' labor practices and history of toxic recalls. Pay attention to the message they're selling through advertising — is sex and underage idealism more on display than the products themselves?

3. **Be a smart shopper.** The cosmetics industry fleeces billions from us every year. Billions. Don't let your vanity make you poor. Spending your rent check at Sephora isn't feminist, it's dumb.

4. **Love yourself with or without the concealer.** We *know* how important concealer is, and neither of us is ashamed to admit

to dabbing it on first thing in the morning even before running for coffee. But work on loving the unaltered version of yourself too — and expect everyone else to do the same.

5. **Don't judge other women based on their beauty habits** — each of us is entitled to be as individual here as she wants to be. If one of your coworkers rocks bleached-blond hair, blue eye shadow, and frosted pink lip gloss, let the woman have her look. If she feels good in her own skin, what do you care? Her individuality is beautiful.

6. **Support women-owned businesses.** We have the power to be selective in all of our purchasing decisions, so when buying beauty products, consider not only your conscience but also other women. Here's where we can help out our sisters without much effort. If you hear about a new beauty company started by a woman in her basement, or by two college friends investing all to follow their dream, consider supporting them.

FIVE

IS DIETING ANTIFEMINIST?

RELATIONSHIPS ARE NO doubt a challenge for modern feminists — we promise, we'll get to that — but the most dysfunctional relationship in many women's lives is the one we have with food. We savor chocolate and champagne with orgasmic delight but punish ourselves for giving in to cravings. Our enthusiasm for cupcakes made them a billion-dollar (and seemingly endless) trend, and yet we feel guilty for eating our own birthday cakes. We're why the Food Network and *The Biggest Loser* exist, and why cookbooks compete with weight-loss books on the bestseller lists. We buy flavorless diet things with bizarre textures and weird aftertastes in an effort to save a few calories a day. We go on diets that consist of just carbs, or no carbs, or just a few carbs, or only brown food, or only raw food, or only French food. We fast, cleanse, and sometimes even endure colonics to feel lighter.

Why can't we just eat normally? The problem, of course, is that women don't see food as just food. It's linked to body size, which is scrutinized by the media and — even more — by us. It's no surprise that nearly eighty million Americans, most of them women, are on diets. There are some legitimate reasons for this: Many of us could certainly stand to eat fewer processed goods and a lot more fresh produce. More than half of our population is considered overweight, and childhood obesity is the new epidemic threatening a generation. A culture that can even think up such phenomena as bacon doughnuts, deep-fried butter, and the Cheesecake Factory doesn't help. But altering what you put in your body so you can live a longer, healthier life is far different than the war most women wage against food. This is a psychological battlefront, and it often begins in early adolescence, sometimes younger. Consider these scary-ass truths:

- Almost half of American children in first, second, and third grades say they want to be thinner.
- 50 percent of nine- and ten-year-old girls say that being on a diet makes them feel better about themselves.
- The rate at which teen girls are taking diet pills nearly doubles every year.
- Between five and ten million women and girls in the United States struggle with eating disorders (one million boys and men do too).

Dieting is one of the most important feminist issues. Susie Orbach's *Fat Is a Feminist Issue* began the conversation three decades ago by suggesting that a woman's weight obsession is not just about being skinny but about having power. A woman's degree of thinness essentially correlates with her ability to succeed in the world. Women are bombarded by messages that "thin equals beautiful" and are held personally responsible — ostracized, scorned, shunned, and ignored — if they don't fit that mold. Sometimes a woman internalizes this and makes dieting a personal power play. Eating is something we have complete control over, and many women use food restriction as a way to take charge of their lives.

Feminist writer and psychotherapist Kim Chernin speculates that women have historically used dieting as a way to compete with men in a man's world. Thinness provides women with the opportunity to mimic the male. Food and weight become the things women can micromanage, Chernin argues in *The Hungry Self: Women, Eating, and Identity*. This focus on the body, of course, masks deeper issues, ones that are magnified by a culture that overvalues external appearance.

The media amplifies this message. "Ads for diets and dieting products, which frequently target females, are based on making women feel shame that there is something wrong with their bodies that can be 'fixed' through dieting," says Judith Matz, a licensed therapist and coauthor of *The Diet Survivor's Handbook: 60 Lessons in Eating, Acceptance, and Self-Care*. The book examines the emotional, physical, and political ramifications of the modern woman's obsession with body size.

"Diets constrict women," Matz says. "On a cultural and political level, the message is that women shouldn't take up too much space. At a physiological level, dieting compromises women's natural ability to regulate their hunger, often leaving them physically uncomfortable from undereating — or from overeating in response to the deprivation caused by diets. Psychologically, with diets comes a preoccupation with food and weight that take up a tremendous amount of mental energy. Where else might women put that energy?"

That energy could certainly power more significant change in women's lives. But is all dieting antifeminist? Are you betraying your gender if you join Weight Watchers or Jenny Craig? It depends on the motivations behind the desire to diet. If the goal is to improve your health and feel good, don't call it dieting; call it living well. If you cite outside influences as motivation — pressure from family, a lover's passing comment about your ass, or a photo of Heidi Klum in *Elle* (you *know* that's altered, right?) — you may not be making the most empowering choice for yourself. We know it's hard. We can't remember a time when food and body image weren't linked to women's self-esteem, including our own. But it's time we break that vicious cycle and learn to love the lady in the mirror.

WOMEN VERSUS WEIGHT: HOW TO STOP THE WAR

Women haven't always been taught to hate food and strive for a slim physique. This phenomenon is quite new, developing within the last few hundred years. Western dieting trends date back to the 1800s, when obesity was first diagnosed as a severe health condition. Doctors recommended dieting to obese patients to combat ailments such as heart disease and strokes. Interestingly, men were the first victims of a new societal ideal that exchanged stout and strong for ripped and rugged — like the Greek gods — to symbolize power, wealth, and worthiness. The female body ideal at the time, however, was valued most when it was Rubenesque, soft, and supple, as this showcased fertility. Thin women were actually criticized in the print media, sometimes called bad mothers and even unpatriotic. Not that we recommend a return to bashing thin girls, of course, but it's clear that ideas about good and bad bodies are societal, not inborn.

In the late 1800s, when Elizabeth Cady Stanton and the first-wave feminists were trying to buck the corset trend, they chose exercise and diet to achieve the hourglass ideal. To them, dieting was the rebellion, not the conformation. *Harper's Bazaar* and other women's magazines of the time condemned the efforts of women to "emancipate themselves through slenderness." In the end, women rejected the corset but not the ideal body shape that was force-fed to them through the media.

And that's just how we're convinced to diet to this day. For as long as the media has been targeting women — pretty much forever — it has been telling us how to live our lives. Or, rather, it has been telling us how to fix everything we're doing wrong — relationships, sex, work, friendship, and exercise and eating. (We realize that in this book, it might seem like we're telling you what to do too, but in fact, we're telling you — for the most part — how to *stop* doing all this stuff you've been told to do. If you want to stop, that is.) Nowadays, being thin is probably the most universally covered of those topics. Every mainstream magazine geared toward women, from *Parenting* to *Playgirl*, has a dieting column. They cover every diet fad as if it were a cultural trend rather than a dangerous manipulation, no matter how bizarre the diet is — the cabbage soup diet, the Zone, Atkins and other "yay, bacon!" fads, the cayenne-pepper-lemonade cleanse, and so on. Thousands of blogs focus on how to lose weight and get thin, and that can be helpful, to a point. Let us again distinguish between healthy weight loss (a good goal) and the fixation with thinness (projecting someone else's idea of healthy/perfect/pretty onto yourself). The former, good; the latter, bad. Got it? Okay.

When feminists criticize dieting today, they're fighting against an image — that "thin equals beautiful" thing again. The dieting industry makes loads preying on women's insecurities — more than $60 billion a year. Its success depends on women feeling like failures, at least as far as their bodies are concerned. Naomi Wolf calls dieting "the most potent political sedative in women's history."

That sedative is injected into our lives via ads that assault us through television, cell phones, e-mail spam, Facebook sidebars, doctor's offices, billboards on highways, signs on subways, and Google searches. Whether they're hawking sneakers or fast food, the ads are effectively selling us the idea that looking like Jennifer Aniston will make us happier (hard to argue against that, right?). A woman can't just throw on sneakers and walk to the mailbox anymore. No, that's for lazy slobs! She needs to lace up "high-performance" shoes that lift and shape her rear end and help her burn calories.

And then there are the images of female bodies that are thrust at us constantly. They're hardly representative of how women actually look. Quick: Name five famous plus-size supermodels. Can't? Okay, who's your favorite fat actress who regularly stars as the lead in romantic comedies? Oh, she doesn't exist; right. And lately even the Kate Moss or Kate Hudson ideal isn't good enough. In 2011, H&M began marketing its clothing on virtual models — plastic mannequins digitally altered to look human, although, with their dislocated-appearing arms and hipbones jutting out of their waists, the models didn't quite achieve that look.

What we find most disturbing is that women today are smart, media-literate, and aware of the bullshit in these campaigns, but nonetheless, so strong is the subconscious mind-fuck in the messages, many women are still buying into it. "We all know that the media is such an incredible force and consumer culture is just designed to make us all feel terrible about our bodies," says Laura Fraser, who chronicled the rise of dieting along with the rise of consumerism (go figure: they're linked) in her book *Losing It: America's Obsession with Weight and the Industry That Feeds on It.* "I think a lot of women are keenly aware of the dichotomy between their philosophies of feminism and the ways they live their lives. That's definitely true with body image. Most of us think it's terrible that we have these skinny models in magazines or skinny actresses on TV but we internalize that we should be like them. Women have an awareness that this body image is oppressive, but it's also the dominant image in our culture and also what our culture has determined is sexy. It really tugs at us."

BREAKING THE SKINNY-IS-SEXY IDEAL

The pressure to be sexy is even stronger than the one to be thin — but make no mistake: you "should" be both. When food and sex mix in advertising, things get confusing. We're tantalized by media imagery that sexualizes food almost as often as we're made to feel guilty for consuming it. A woman's relationship with food as portrayed in commercials is bipolar: She's either ordering the salad and barely picking at it or dripping barbecue sauce down her exposed, perpetually moist cleavage while writhing on the hood of a car. The barbecue sauce also gives her an orgasm, of course. This pornification of food has been most prevalent in Carl's Jr. ads in the past decade: Paris Hilton making out with her burger in a ridiculously complicated peekaboo swimsuit while washing a car (the logistics here are mind-boggling). Reality star Audrina Patridge in a gold bikini sucking on the pineapple from her teriyaki burger. Kim Kardashian making out with a salad on her bed — and then in the bathtub. *Gawker* coined the term *slutburger* to describe this genre of television commercial.

What's being sold, other than the burgers, is the message that women can pig out on food but only if they can be sexy while doing it — and only if they're hot enough to turn men on. Larger women need not apply. When the company is confronted with the obvious bias in its commercials' casting (which happens about every time a new slutburger ad airs), its response is always the same: Carl's Jr. is selling burgers to young men. Got that, ladies? No meat for you! The assumption here is that big, juicy burgers are for men only. Women shouldn't be eating such stuff — just, you know, dripping it on their half-naked bodies.

If sexy food commercials are for men, weight-loss ads are certainly for women. However, looking at the campaigns for the country's biggest diet chains, we see sex being sold here too. For example, Jenny Craig employs actresses and pop stars to transform themselves from slightly above average weight to bikini-body skinny. This is more problematic than it might seem at first glance. When our few prominent cultural models of bodies that aren't unnaturally thin constantly harp on their new-and-improved status, it takes away their power. That translates, subtly, into a message that the size they were before was *not okay*. And then, if these spokesmodels can't go full-waif and keep it that way, they're criticized for it. (Kirstie Alley, we love you because you're funny, period.) Jenny pawn Mariah Carey did a 2011 ad for the company that consisted of her breaking through black silk — OMG, she *is* a butterfly — and showcasing her "Jenny body," taut new tummy on full display. Not only was Carey a world-renowned superstar (with the means to employ a team of health and fitness professionals, and don't think for one second that she didn't), but she'd given birth to twins less than a year before this ad was shot. Subtext: Even new moms who have twins can get rock-hard abs again. But what if, maybe, they can't? And what if women sometimes can't lose that last ten pounds they have on their weight-loss-program goal sheets, make stretch marks disappear, or banish cellulite? That's the problem with our diet-obsessed culture. It pressures women to constantly struggle for unattainable perfection — or at least to be a few pounds lighter, and then a few more pounds.

These ads also sell a skewed sense of sisterhood. On weight-loss commercials, women are often shown celebrating, as if losing twenty pounds were the greatest achievement of a woman's life. Sometimes losing weight can be a victory — if you've escaped life-threatening obesity, for example — but we'd wager motherhood, a career accomplishment, learning a second language, or any number of other triumphs would be even better. Chernin argues that what these women are really celebrating is being in control. "What unites the women who seek to reduce their weight is the fact that they look for an answer to their life's problems in the control of their bodies and appetites," she wrote. "A woman who walks through the doors of a weight-watching organization and enters the women's reduction movement has allowed her culture to persuade her that significant relief from her personal and cultural dilemma is to be found in the reduction of her body. Thus, her decision, although she may not be aware of it, enters the domain of the body politic and becomes symbolically a political act."

DIETING WHILE FEMINIST

So it's clear that dieting (as opposed to sensible healthy eating) is evil, right? But women still do it. Cut yourself some slack and know you're in good company. There seems to be an unfortunate inevitability that most women will try to control their body size by fighting food at some time in their lives.

Feminist Confessions: Lessons Learned from Dieting

I'm brand-new to dieting — I just took it up a few weeks ago, after discovering I'd gained ten pounds in the past six months or so. What's funny is I still hate admitting this, not because I'm embarrassed to have gained weight, but because I've never had to deal with it before. Mine is the naturally thin body type that provokes disparaging remarks like "Eat a cookie!" rather than "Stop eating that cookie!" — still insulting. Now, the neuroses we all have surrounding body issues is such that I feel guilty for not having needed a diet before! And yet, when I then tell my boyfriend I don't want to go to the new grilled-cheese restaurant for fear of blowing my diet, I hate how that sounds too! (I may have even uttered the evil words "I'm sorry I'm being such a girl about this." Ugh, I'm so sorry, feminism!)

The good news, however, is that I feel I chose the right time to gain ten pounds, because there is a wonderful invention at my disposal: the dieting app. My sister recommended MyFitnessPal to me with the fervor of a zealot, and I now understand why. It allows the easiest calorie-counting in recorded history: You simply type in what you ate, and it automatically calculates the calories. Or, if you don't even feel like typing, you can scan the bar codes on prepackaged goods. I doubt I ever would have counted calories the old-fashioned way, but now I'm instantly aware of my intake at all times, as well as the subtractions made for workouts.

Through using this app, I've realized that I may have gained this weight simply by eating as much as my boyfriend does at our dinners out, which probably come more frequently than is healthy. (I had developed more elaborate theories about birth control pills and antidepressants, which may in fact be contributing, but the truth is I need to stay on both of those, so calorie-counting it is.) One of my favorite things about this app is that it scolds you if you don't eat enough: Drop below 1,200 net calories in a day, and it'll explain to you why that's not helping anyone. This, if nothing else, soothes my feminist heart. Another wonderful development: My tech-geek boyfriend saw my app and liked it so much — "It's like a game!" he said — that he got it, too, and "friended" me instantly. Now we're counting calories together, and neither of us has to bemoan feeling "like a girl."

— *Jennifer Keishin Armstrong*

My dieting history is totally cliché and utterly unfeminist. I was a teenage dancer-cum-anorexic. I tried half a dozen fad diets and as many cleanses, and I regularly embarked on extreme workout regimens to prep for things like the beginning of a school year or a wedding. I actually can't remember a time after adolescence when I wasn't on some form of diet or weight-loss mission. I know; this all sucks for my feminist cred. So I was shocked when the one event in my life that I expected would throw my body image into disarray turned out to be the thing that made me chill out and stop dieting altogether. I got pregnant, gained forty pounds, and stopped obsessing.

To be truthful, it took some time and serious hard work to get my mental health in check. When I first stopped fitting in my regular clothes, I freaked out. I knew that was coming, but it happened at around four months, when I didn't really have a baby bump yet; I was just a little bigger everywhere. I remember envying women clearly in their third trimesters — it's impossible not to look adorable with a baby bump, no matter what you wear. I wanted that key accessory instead of just bigger thighs and boobs. When my bump finally came, I embraced it. I wore form-fitting dresses, leggings with slender tunics, and bikinis. I felt beautiful, mostly because I was so proud of the little life, now clearly showcased, causing all these changes. And dieting? Obviously: no. Not just because it's unhealthy to restrict your food intake too much while pregnant (deadly, even), but also because I wanted to eat better than I ever had before — healthy, wholesome, delicious food — and as much of it as I needed.

When I gave birth and was left with the extra weight, sans adorable bump, I slipped into the darkness for a bit. I knew I couldn't diet because I was committed to breastfeeding, but I did think about it (a lot) and found myself turning down some of the baked goods our friends and family so lovingly brought to us during those first weeks. The truth is, person-making takes a major toll on your body, and there are moments when it's just plain terrifying to face the fact that you have changed forever.

Months passed, I eased back into working out, I kept up the calorie-blasting breastfeeding, and the pounds melted away. So too did my obsession with the size and shape I thought I needed to be. Nearly a year later (that's the average time it takes a healthy, noncelebrity woman to lose all her baby weight, by the way) I'm about ten pounds heavier than my pre-baby weight. And guess what: I'm cool with those ten pounds. Really. I know to get them off and keep them off, I'd have to go on a diet of some sort and kick up my exercise routine, make it a daily event instead of the when-I-can-get-to-it activity it is now. I could do it, but I don't really want to. I would rather buy bigger jeans than take time away from my family to hit the gym every day. And I don't want to stop eating carbs. Carbs are fucking good. I am healthy and happy, which is the feminist diet I've needed all along.

— Heather Wood Rudúlph

Eve Ensler, one of the most vocal feminist activists around, got women to love their vaginas through her V-Day campaign and the now-classic *Vagina Monologues*, but even she couldn't escape the pressure to hate herself. She took on women's loathing for their bodies in her book *The Good Body*, a project that grew from her own suffocating self-judgment. "The pattern of the perfect body

has been programmed into me since birth," she wrote. "But whatever the cultural influences and pressures, my preoccupation with
my flab, my constant dieting, exercising, worrying, is self-imposed.
I pick up the magazines. *I* buy into the ideal. *I* believe that blond,
flat girls have the secret. What is far more frightening than narcis-
sism is the zeal for self-mutilation that is spreading, infecting the
world."

Oprah always knows how to help *us*, but she spent her entire
life not understanding how to have her own healthy relationship
with food. After years of public weight battles — and essentially being the face of women's dieting struggles — Oprah came to terms
with her own insecurities and shared this aha moment: "The
choices we make about what we put in our mouths are only stand-
ins for the beliefs we carry in our minds and our hearts." We have
to learn to love ourselves before we can love pie — and we should
love pie!

Whether you've had this epiphany or still classify a sweet or
salty delicacy as a cheat (cheating on what, exactly?), you are part
of helping women break this cycle of food (and self-) hatred. Even
tiny steps in a more healthy, self-loving direction can help this all-
too-important feminist cause.

Sexy Feminist Action Plan: Developing a Healthy Association with Food

Giving up all dieting is drastic, especially if it's almost always
been a part of your life. Many of us can't remember a time when
food intake wasn't governed by a personal goal, health experi-

ment, or fitness plan. Learning how to eat without a negative food association could take years. So instead of giving up all control of your food, make small but critical moves to understand your relationship with the things you eat. We should care more about eating healthy, unprocessed foods that make us feel good than about calorie count.

1. If you're going to diet, set positive goals for yourself and be encouraging. Your intention should be to feel better, not to fit into something better.

2. Embrace women of all shapes and sizes, even the gal downing a Whopper while you're on a juice cleanse. (Question: Do you really need to be on a juice cleanse?)

3. Don't give in to fads. Atkins, the Zone, South Beach, celebrity miracle diets: There will always be a new supposed wonder cure that promises to help you "shed pounds instantly." Know that if something sounds too good to be true, it definitely is. We've heard it over and over again, but it bears repeating: The only way to improve your health and lose weight is to eat more whole foods and fewer processed foods and to exercise regularly — and responsibly. We all know this by now, so let's follow our intuition already. Besides, it can only help women overall to make the diet industry — that is, the fat-shaming industry — less lucrative.

4. When you begin a new exercise routine — whether it's training for a marathon, going rock climbing, or doing power yoga, all of which require you to use your body in ways you haven't before — consult your doctor, not just about the obvious physical health risks but about the proper calories you

should be consuming. Extreme exercise plus dieting is not a quick way to lose weight; it could be a quick way to wind up in the ER. You might also end up burning muscle instead of fat, negating your efforts anyway.

5. Use food as food, not as an emotional bargaining chip. Denying yourself dessert one night because you were "bad" the night before only reinforces a negative relationship to the food you obviously love and crave. It's not bad to eat cake. Just don't eat the whole damn thing. Conversely, food shouldn't be a reward for accomplishing tasks or being good for a week.

6. Eat what you want. This sounds simple and somewhat naïve, but if you don't enjoy your food, you're missing the whole point. Duh moment: Obviously you need to have a healthy overall diet, understand what portion control means, and avoid anything that affects you negatively. You're the only one in control of what goes in your mouth. Own that responsibility.

SIX

BEING A FASHIONISTA *CAN* BE EMPOWERING

EMINISM AND FASHION have a storied history, and it's more than just the relationship a certain wave of feminists had with their bras. Sometimes the fashions have been oppressive (burqas), other times downright painful (corsets). But there have also been moments of triumph that helped women gain serious feminist ground (pants and business suits). Empowerment in fashion today means reconciling the lengths to which we go to feel glamorous without compromising our health, happiness, and self-esteem.

Fashion is also a fun, freeing expression of individuality. Women can decorate and adorn themselves with exotic, beautiful textiles and accessories to create unique, powerful images. And anyone who's ever found the perfect pair of jeans (stretch denim just may be the greatest invention of our lifetimes) knows that fashion can also be a major self-esteem booster.

But sometimes living la vida fashionista can hurt. Women cram their feet into too small, too tall shoes; wrap their midsections in Lycra to fit into jeans or skirts; and give in to trends that elicit either pain or pangs of embarrassment by distorting their bodies — and body images. Ask any woman about the horrors of the dressing room or about never, ever being able to find jeans that fit, and the fashion industry's biggest failure is revealed. It still caters to one body type; plus-size clothing lines often seem to be poorly constructed afterthoughts. *Project Runway* star Tim Gunn took designers to task for ignoring larger women in a 2011 *Marie Claire* interview. He said, "It's horrifying. Whoever's designing for plus-size doesn't get it. . . . You can't just take a size 8 and make it larger." He added, "Most [designers] say, 'I don't want a woman who's a size 10 or 11 wearing my clothes.' Well, shame on you! It's not realistic. We need to address real women with real needs." Oh, Tim. We wish you lived in our closets and gave us morning pep talks. But even more, we wish this weren't such a glaring problem. The physical and emotional pain caused by some kinds of clothing inhibit a woman's ability to use fashion as a form of feminist expression. But we think we can get past that.

FASHION'S FEMINIST — AND SOMETIMES NOT SO FEMINIST — HISTORY

Women have been using style to express their attitudes, femininity, and personalities for centuries. Clothing has also historically been used to oppress women, restrict their options in society, and keep them confined to second-class citizenship. From this history, fashion's feminist power was discovered. Some of our most significant milestones:

Corsets. These must-have accessories (for centuries!) were torture mechanisms. The cages — once made of steel — constricted women's midsections to the extent that skeletal deformity and internal-organ damage were common female medical problems. If there were any question about whether they were purposely used to enslave women to fashion, we offer this quote from a Victorian-era man: "If you want a girl to grow up gentle and womanly in her ways and her feelings, lace her tight." Parisian visionaries in the 1900s loosened the suffocating strings when haute couture was invented and creativity branched beyond asphyxiating women. Coco Chanel led the charge. She revolutionized fashion by toning down the popular dramatic aesthetic of the early 1900s and offering women casual, comfortable clothes. She also made a name for herself by stating that women should dress for themselves, not husbands, lovers, or bosses. Being able to breathe became a new priority for women.

The corset remains a style staple in fashion even today, albeit in a much more tame version. When it's not crushing ribs, a corset is damn sexy, bringing attention to a woman's waist and lifting her breasts. There's power in that sexuality. Madonna knew it (think the Blond Ambition world tour and those ridiculous/fabulous Jean Paul Gaultier corsets paired with men's trousers). Today the likes of Rihanna, Beyoncé, and Lady Gaga know it too — their sexy/edgy costumes walk the line between overexposed and empowering. Because their music skews toward the latter, and their attitude makes their intentions clear — they are no one's objectified pawns — we support this use of sexuality as weaponry.

But we wonder if they'd wear pants more (or ever) if they knew how hard early feminists fought for the right to wear them.

Pants. Fashion's feminist hero Coco Chanel had a hand in introducing women to this garment, which was previously off-limits to ladies — first by law, then mostly by custom. Chanel's trousers were comfortable, functional, and chic. They made everyday activities such as riding a horse, caring for children, and even walking less cumbersome.

Cut to the denim revolution of the 1980s, which eventually led to the technology that gave us perfectly tailored designer jeans. Goodbye, mom jeans and cardboard-textured Levi's! While the price tag on many of these styles could be prohibitory ($250, really?), the demand for jeans that finally — finally — made everyone's ass look good caused an influx of them in the industry. Soon even mass-market retailers were carrying them. And today, almost every woman can find a pair of jeans she feels good in.

Miniskirts. Shorter skirts initially came about out of necessity rather than fashion. In the 1940s, materials were scarce due to World War II, and women had fewer textiles to work with. If a woman wanted a new skirt, she had to make it a shorter one. The 1950s brought the boring-housewife aesthetic, so the young women of the 1960s wanted a revolution, and the miniskirt became a feminist's secret weapon. The signature mini-dresses of the sixties didn't come from Paris or even New York Fashion Week but from youths in cities across America rebelling against the image of the ideal woman: the happy homemaker who didn't speak — or shop — for herself.

Fashion designers tried to force a miniskirt revival, along with a resurgence of all things feminine, on unwilling female shoppers in the 1980s, as Susan Faludi documents in her groundbreaking book *Backlash: The Undeclared War Against American Women.* "'Going soft' doesn't have to mean losing your edge," Saks Fifth Avenue ads told women, assuring them they could wear the new, more feminine styles. Magazines argued that embracing girlie fashion instead of suits was feminist, because it showed that femininity was valued in the workplace. However, a 1988 *New York Times*/CBS News poll found that only a quarter of adult women had worn a skirt above the knee even once in the previous year. "I will wear the new short skirts when men wear rompers to the office," *Working Woman* columnist Kathleen Fury wrote. NPR legal-affairs reporter Nina Totenberg told female listeners, "Hold the line. Don't buy. And the mini will die." The fashion industry gave in the next season, adding more pantsuits and longer skirts to their lines. What women wanted won out . . . for a while.

Whether because women finally gave in to industry pressures or because a younger generation of up-and-coming lady executives simply had different ideas about work wear, miniskirts returned to power in the 1990s. In popular culture, TV characters such as Amanda Woodward on *Melrose Place* and the hot lady lawyers of *Ally McBeal* embodied a new sexy-bitch image. These women were definitely not afraid to show off their legs in their miniskirted power suits, and millions of their young viewers followed their lead. The authors of this book were among them, though we hardly thought of it as a feminist statement at the time.

Menswear for women. The 1970s, of course, was the decade of what people most easily recognize as the modern feminist movement. The fight was as heated as ever, and feminists took their physical images as seriously as their political views. Miniskirts and body-hugging outfits were abandoned for a masculine aesthetic that made men see the person, not her boobs or thighs. High-profile idols of empowerment such as Diane Keaton and Gloria Steinem showed that muted tones, bell-bottoms, and masculine blazers could be items of coveted beauty.

An offshoot of this trend was the rise in androgynous fashion. Women experimented with their masculinity using garments that neither defined nor hid their feminine assets. This staple of gay culture found a new place in the zeitgeist. Gender-bending was the new sexy, and it turned us on. Models Jenny Shimizu and, later, Agyness Deyn became It girls for walking the masculine/feminine line. Serbian Australian model Andrej Pejic became one of the most in-demand models in 2010 for his stunning, androgynous beauty. He walked in both men's and women's haute couture shows and made headlines in 2011 for appearing in a German ad for a push-up bra. And transsexual model Lea T landed the cover of *Elle Brazil* in December 2011.

Sexy Feminist: Lady Gaga

Most talk about Lady Gaga concerns what she's wearing, be it a tangled web of barbed wire or a dress made out of meat. But we're more enamored with what she's saying with her extreme wardrobe. Through fashion, she has protested the use of fur (an outfit made from dozens of stuffed Kermit dolls), told the world she was *not* a piece of meat (that steak suit), and riffed on how society mutes women (all those lacy facemasks circa "Bad Romance"). She says of most of her outfit choices, "They're meant to be kind of a rejection of what people view about women. . . . I am a feminist. And I want to change the way people view women." She went on to say she wasn't interested "in being a perfect placid pop singer that looks great in bikinis."

Her visual art also works as activism in a way not even Madonna could pull off. In 2011, she opened the MTV Video Music Awards singing as her alter ego Jo Calderone, whom she identifies as a transgender man. That act, and her song "Born This Way," allowed gender identity to become a part of mainstream discussion. There have been a lot of pro-gay celebrity icons, but few have put their names and fame on the line to fight for change the way Gaga has. When rampant bullying led to a string of gay suicides in 2011, Gaga stormed Capitol Hill and demanded legislation to promote tolerance. The same year, she practically stalked President Obama, finally confronting him at a campaign rally to urge the repeal of Don't Ask, Don't Tell. When the measure to kill the policy finally passed, later that year, celebration rallies played Lady Gaga songs on loudspeakers.

She's been equally vocal about women's rights and humanitarian issues. Her Monster Ball tour raised more than $80,000 for homeless youth. When an earthquake hit Haiti in 2010, she staged a special concert and donated every dollar — more than $500,000 — to relief efforts. And when Gaga became one of the latest faces of MAC's VIVA Glam line, in 2011, she did more than just pose in the gorgeous pictorials and give journalists another opportunity to ask her about her wardrobe. Alongside feminist pop royalty Cyndi Lauper, Gaga went on the talk-show circuit armed with stunning knowledge of the issues, spouting statistics about women's HIV infection rates and emphasizing the urgency for girlfriends to tell one another to be sexually responsible. "We want women to feel strong and feel strong enough that they can remember to protect themselves. To have this lipstick as a reminder in your purse, that when your man is laying naked in bed, you go into the bathroom, you put your lipstick on, and you bring a condom out with you. There are no exceptions."

The spectacle of Lady Gaga would be just spectacle without the strong-armed messages she insists on shoving in the world's face: be kind, respect women, celebrate equality, and love yourself.

Stilettos. Heels have been used throughout history as tools of oppression and symbols of wealth and status. The modern stiletto was invented in the 1950s and still causes controversy: Can feminists walk proudly in four-inch heels? While the shoe named after a deadly weapon and popularized through porn (hi again!) has its oppressive origins, wearing heels today doesn't feel like a feminist betrayal. There are myriad options for fabulous shoes for women, so if a gal prefers the leg-toning effects of Jimmy Choos, more power to her. Plus, if she has the earning power to afford four-hundred-dollar shoes, that's progress worth celebrating.

Lingerie. Underthings have come a long way. Early lingerie was ugly and uncomfortable — bloomers bigger than modern cargo shorts; cone-shaped bras with straps as wide as seat belts. Much of this was due to the stigma that classified lingerie as scandalous. As if accepting that stigma as a challenge, lingerie designers in the twentieth century invested as much in technological break-throughs to lift, separate, shape, and flatter as they did in creating a sexy silhouette.

This, of course, became a feminist problem. The rise in sexy undergarments was considered to be yet another way for men to fetishize women, define their value based solely on their sexual-ity, and profit, once again, from women's body insecurities. While there's no doubt the porn aesthetic is all over lingerie advertising, ladies are benefiting from modern lingerie too. Thongs may seem to be more about sex than function, but many women feel more comfortable in them and like not having to worry about panty lines. Bras encrusted in diamonds are both dumb and obviously just titillating toys for men (while paying lip service to the gross "diamonds are a girl's best friend" concept), but modern (normal) bras are magic. Yes, magic. Ask a woman about her favorite bra and she'll ooze excitement about how it has changed her life. She didn't spend fifty dollars on an undergarment constructed by engi-neers to feel exploited. Boob management is an important skill, no matter their size.

THE FEMINISM IN FASHION: FINDING YOUR OWN SENSE OF STYLE

Whether you die for your miniskirts or prefer the comfy slacks of Lands' End, you are being fashion-feminist if you are defining your own sense of style. That act itself is a little bit badass. Fashion at its core is rebellious. Think of subculture trends such as goth, hippie, and hipster. These terms describe lifestyles as much as they do looks, and that's fashion at its best. Fashion gives subcultures an opportunity to define themselves and demand to be recognized. The rise in queer fashion, fat fashion, and cultural clothing reflects groups demanding to be heard — and dressing to be noticed.

Fashion also gives women a chance to use their sexuality as political power. The women of the Riot Grrrl movement took traditionally girlie garments such as baby-doll dresses and cropped shirts and wore them ripped, paired with black leather, and vandalized with graffitied words such as *slut* and *rape*. Along with the music that lashed out at rape culture, racism, and patriarchy, the image had a definite impact.

Madonna is the master at using fashion as a political statement. Her various incarnations — from virgin/whore bride to sleek dominatrix — were deliberately explicit. She used herself as a billboard for female sexuality, calling attention to it rather than allowing society to exploit her. Not everyone got it. Fashion designer Bob Mackie once said of Madonna's most iconic imagery: "That Madonna look was vulgar. It was overly sexually expressive. The slits and the clothes cut up and pulled all around; you couldn't tell the sluts from the schoolgirls." Bob, *that* was the *point*.

The fact that "schoolgirl" is one of the most sexualized images in modern culture is part of the problem. Young girls today are influenced not by style icons such as Coco Chanel and Kathleen Hanna, but by MTV. A teen or tween girl is at the cusp of forming her identity. Imagine if she'd never seen fashion magazines or MTV, especially now that it's the network of drunk-girls-in-minimal-clothing reality television. Would she dress more authentically like herself rather than marching into first period wearing the skinny jeans and tight tops that are selling at Forever 21?

A young girl's sense of self is often directly linked to her fashion sense. The more authentic and un-stifled her experience growing up (and the more positive female role models she has), the more creative her sense of style is likely to be. Take, for example, budding fashion icon and publishing wunderkind Tavi Gevinson. At age eleven, she was blogging about Commes des Garçons and Rodarte with the type of fervor most girls that age reserve for their latest teen heartthrob crush. By age sixteen, Tavi was running RookieMag.com, a website for teens that addresses issues from boy woes to what feminism means for girls today and does it with wit, wisdom, and age-appropriate enthusiasm. For her, fashion obsession, feminism, and homework are equally important. She painstakingly pairs thrift-store clothes with haute couture to create a look that is at once girlie and totally punk rock. She interviews Gloria Steinem. She says "ugh" a lot. She's a teenager who's comfortable in her own skin — and clothes. Every girl, teen, and woman deserves to find herself this way.

Feminist Confessions: How I Found Myself Through Fashion

I wasn't a big fashion girl growing up — my clothing-related memories from my teens involve mainly the Guess jeans, leggings, and oversize sweaters of the '80s and '90s, the mega-trends that told people nothing more about me than that I lived in the mall culture of my time. I slid downward from there, living in sweats throughout college. When I entered the work force, I traded in my leggings and sweaters for pretending-to-be-a-grownup cheap skirt suits, beige slacks, and button-down blouses.

This didn't change until I moved to New York, started working for a national magazine, and suddenly found myself. And the self I found did *not* wear slacks. I realized I needed to change my life drastically when I saw a photo of myself: I was wearing a pastel-striped sweater and polyester-blend slacks from Express, and I had a bobbed haircut with blond highlights in my naturally brown hair. I looked not far from how my mom looked in what she now refers to as her "mom phase" of dressing — like a girl trying to be a woman by wearing incredibly lame clothes. I now refer to that time as "when I was a desperate housewife" — because that's what I saw in that photo, which was taken while I was living with my fiancé in the New Jersey suburbs.

Once I broke off my engagement, at age thirty, and moved into my own tiny apartment in Manhattan's East Village, I knew a fashion change was immediately in order. I entered what I think of as my hot-pink phase: I owned a pink trench coat, a pink cargo skirt, a pink messenger bag, pink stiletto boots, and black sandals adorned with buckles and lined with, you guessed it, pink. I can't imagine what this phase was about. One can assume it had something to do with expressing my femininity, or maybe even a much-delayed adolescence. Luckily, I eventually saw that I was attracted mostly to the cargo skirt, messenger bag, and sandals, and that I could do without the pink-washing. At the same time, I got way into classic chick-rock, and my real transformation began: I stared at photos of Joan Jett and Pat Benatar to copy their looks. I dyed my hair black and got blunt bangs cut. I shifted from pink to black.

Through this process, I discovered other fashion role models, such as French singer/fashion royalty Charlotte Gainsbourg, who favors a girlier rock look, as if Audrey Hepburn fronted a band. (Yes, this is why I swoon for her.) Now, as I find myself shifting into yet another phase of my life — more settled, thanks to my boyfriend and my general exhaustion with going out, and more introspective and artsy, thanks to my looming book deadlines — I've even rediscovered one of my original fashion icons, Rhoda of *The Mary Tyler Moore Show*, played by the gorgeous Valerie Harper. I'm integrating her graphic scarves and flowy fabrics into my look and loving it.

More than anything, though, I'm loving the chance to channel women whose essences I want to incorporate into my own with the simple choice of what I put on every day. I don't think it's any coincidence that I chose strong, undeniably feminist women as my fashion icons; Joan, Pat, Charlotte, and Rhoda have helped me find the rocking, feminine, artsy woman inside of me.

— Jennifer Keishin Armstrong

Sexy Feminist Action Plan: Making Fashion Feminist

The key, of course, is to make fashion your own. There's nothing feminist in copying everyone else or buying what you think is trendy if it makes you feel awkward, exploited, or just plain weird. Remember that, at its core, fashion is communication. Here's your opportunity to express your individuality every time you open your closet.

1. Sexy doesn't have to be slutty. The female body is a beautiful, wondrous thing — you are supposed to love it and feel proud showing it off. Wear *whatever* makes you feel great, no matter what anyone tells you. But if you're having trouble figuring out what makes you feel good, we'll tell you our own guideline for feeling sexy without feeling overexposed: When in doubt, showcase (hell, flaunt) one asset — back, navel, legs, cleavage, arms, clavicle — but only one at a time. This practice often yields the most dramatic, memorable results. Think about the difference between the sheer navel-revealing Versace gown Jennifer Lopez wore to the 2000 Grammy Awards and the long-sleeved, backless Guy Laroche gown Hilary Swank wore to the 2005 Oscars. Both made headlines, but for different reasons. J-Lo's dress was marveled at for staying on — and barely concealing all of her naughty bits. Hilary's was the standout look of the red-carpet season for daring to reveal . . . less. Don't forget that fashion is a way to show the world who you feel you really are, but you don't necessarily have to show all of you.

2. **Wear what fits.** Fashion clearly skews skinny, and not every style you see on the pages of your favorite women's glossy is going to look good on you — in fact, most won't. So try on clothes and purchase what you feel comfortable in. If it pinches, flattens, or interferes with your ability to move normally, you're probably wearing the wrong size. And by trying to squeeze yourself into a size or style you think you should be wearing, you're likely doing your natural figure a disservice. Similarly, if you're hiding in clothes that are too big or boxy, liberate your lovely body! Stylist and wardrobe-makeover queen Stacy London put it best: "I feel very

strongly that style is about the individual, not the industry. . . . If you use yourself as the lens, you are absolutely going to look better than if you try to mimic some 40-foot billboard of a model who's retouched and 12 years old."

3. **Don't bankrupt yourself in the name of fashion.** Couture pieces are beautiful works of art and rightfully command thousands for their unique, handmade details. But some labels add extra zeros to their price tags just for status. Don't be a sucker. Splurge on long-lasting investment pieces (a trench coat, wear-daily designer jeans, a little black dress). Buy your everyday staples (the garments that are most frequently replaced) for cheap.

4. **Shop consciously.** Shopping while feminist takes a little research. It's easy to scoop up armloads of cheap T-shirts at places like American Apparel and Walmart. But know where your money goes when you're buying from each retailer. (We talk more about this important issue in the afterword.) And, of course, stop supporting any store or clothing line that treats women badly in their advertising.

SEVEN

THE WORKING-WOMAN PROBLEM

A WALL STREET SECRETARY with big hair, high heels, and a Staten Island accent has a brilliant idea for a merger deal, but her sleek, shoulder-padded female boss hogs the credit for it. Only a chance skiing accident that lays up the evil Katharine Parker (Sigourney Weaver) for several weeks can provide salvation for poor Tess McGill (Melanie Griffith) — who uses the opportunity to pretend she's the boss, grab the credit she deserves, and (bonus!) steal the bitch's boyfriend too.

Working Girl was touted as a tale of female empowerment, but of course, Tess succeeded only by, as Susan Faludi's *Backlash* pointed out, "playing the daffy and dependent girl." Worse, her empowerment came at the expense of another, more powerful woman. *But*, you protest, *that was way back in 1988! We've progressed since then, right? Women aren't still fighting each other for power, influence, and men's attention in offices both fictionalized and real, are they?* Alas, more than ever: "As more and more women have flooded into the workplace, it's gotten to be a bigger problem, just because there are more of us," says Nan Mooney, whose 2005 book *I Can't Believe She Did That!* tracked why women tend to betray each other at work. "I think it really stems from a lot of the lessons we learn as children, that women should be good, that we should avoid conflict. Now we have to be achievers, but without ever stepping on anyone's toes."

The ironic result? Passive-aggressive baiting and emotional manipulation instead of straightforward confrontation. "Little girls," Mooney adds, "get to be very skilled in relational aggression, where you use relationships against each other as opposed to hitting each other in the face." That's not, we should note, because women are simply born that way; we're taught such skills by parents, authority figures, and movies like *Working Girl.*

Case in point: Even our beloved more-feminist-than-not *30 Rock* offered an example of a subtler, more modern *Working Girl*–like office dilemma in a 2011 plot line that highlighted women's confused attitudes about female coworkers. In it, our heroine Liz Lemon (Tina Fey) hires Abby, a hot new female comic, to join the staff of her comedy show, *TGS*, after Liz is accused of sexism by the (fictional) website JoanofSnark.com. Emphasis on *hot*, because Abby's act seems to involve mostly blond pigtails, tight T-shirts, short-shorts, knee socks, and a baby-soft voice. The guys around the office love it; spotlight-hogging *TGS* star Jenna Maroney (Jane Krakowski) hates it. Liz hates it, too, though for different reasons than Jenna. She tries to teach Abby about feminism and digs up an old video of Abby with brown hair, minimal makeup, modest attire, and a normal voice. When Liz leaks the video online, she learns a lesson. It's revealed that Abby adopted her fake personality to hide from an abusive stalker, and now Abby's forced to quit. We're left to ponder whether Liz was right or wrong to fight Abby's bimbo persona in the first place. Fey herself seems to think Liz might have been wrong, given what she tells us in her book *Bossypants*. "My unsolicited advice to women in the workplace is this," she writes. "When faced with sexism or ageism or lookism or even really aggressive Buddhism, ask yourself the following question: 'Is this person in between me and what I want to do?' If the answer is no, ignore it and move on. Your energy is better used doing your work and outpacing people that way. Then, when you're in charge, don't hire the people who were jerky to you."

Both of these examples are, of course, simply pop-culture depictions of office life, but they bring up — and reinforce — a problem we've heard even the most feminist women whisper about with guilt. When it comes to careers, women have come a long way in the last forty years or so. We still don't make what men do, but we're taking up more seats at the boardroom tables than we used to and we've made great strides in terms of sexual-harassment awareness. But the deep, dark secret is this: many women still have a hard time working with other women.

THE PROBLEM: INFIGHTING FOR ADVANCEMENT DOESN'T HELP ANYBODY

Talk about the glass ceiling all you'd like — don't worry, it's still there, even with its occasional cracks — but women are often taught to erect glass walls among themselves in the workplace. But the only way we can attain real equality is to notice the ways our culture divides us and to unite against those insidious currents. We might not be able to wake up in the morning and put *reverse the wage gap* on our to-do lists. (How is that still *here?*) One thing we can do in our everyday lives, however, is help one another out and up as much as possible. But as the two examples from pop culture above illustrate, that's not easy. Katharine's under pressure as a female leader on Wall Street *in the 1980s*, and then here comes this secretary who *hasn't* paid her dues trying to leapfrog over her? (Not to mention the Harrison Ford–stealing.) And Abby on *30 Rock* could've been up to any number of things — co-opting female stereotypes for humor, using her looks to get ahead (in entertainment, go figure!) — even with that stalker twist. In both cases, the women got under each other's professional skins for one reason: because they were women vying for spots in the same male-dominated worlds, and they'd been conditioned to think they were in direct competition with only each other instead of with their male colleagues too.

Hence the girl-on-girl infighting. A 2009 study by the Workplace Bullying Institute found that women who verbally abuse and sabotage their cohorts aim their bile at other women more than 70 percent of the time, while male offenders target both genders equally. The fact is, taking down other women in the workplace *can* work in your short-term professional favor — otherwise, women wouldn't keep doing it so much. It is, to some degree, an unfortunate side effect of well-intentioned affirmative-action programs — if only one woman can get the token-female spot, it follows that all women are in competition with one another for it. And, well, it's not hard to see the upside of male bosses: They're more likely to fall prey to our female charms. They're more likely to promote a woman just to show how un-sexist they are. They're more likely to be easy on us out of some kind of daddy-savior-macho complex. We'd rather rise in the ranks without relying on our femininity — and certainly don't support women who use their sexuality as a workplace bargaining chip — but this is a war; most of us will take any victory we can get.

"A lot of people think [infighting] is a thing of the past, from when women were just breaking in, but as women get higher up, there's more pressure, and they feel more insecure about their positions," Mooney says. "They feel threatened by anyone coming up behind them who's skilled because it feels like there's not that much space at the top. They also feel they better make damn sure that no one messes up underneath them. It's a lot of pressure." To be sure, this is hardly just a problem trumped up by pop-culture depictions of women in the workplace. California-based leadership coach Peggy Klaus has observed the same thing, time and again, with women often offering the same excuse for taking down their female coworkers: "Why help someone who could replace you?"

Women in leadership positions fare even worse in their employees' eyes. A Gallup Poll in 2006 found women still prefer having a male boss. Friends of ours complain of female higher-ups who can't tell the difference between "boss" and "bestie": "I once worked on two massive projects at the same time, both shepherded by the same female boss," says one midlevel professional who declined to be identified. "She was such a nightmare, because when she wasn't needling me about every possible detail about the projects, she'd over-share about her problems with her boyfriend. I tried to hide from her in the subway once. She found me. Talked my ear off about the boyfriend." Others swear female bosses have campaigned to get them fired and demeaned their work at the office, only to turn on the warm charm outside its walls.

We're not trying to blame the victims here — sexism still runs rampant in too many fields, and that's not our fault as women. Careers in law enforcement, the military, and the clergy are still often difficult or impossible for women. They're troublesome enough that they have their own terms: *brass ceiling* for military and law enforcement ranks; *stained-glass ceiling* for religious leadership. But that's why it's so important for us to get to the top without taking one another down.

A History of the Working Woman — and Her Competitive Urges — in Pop Culture

1942: Rosie the Riveter becomes a symbol of the women who took over the factories and kept America productive while the men headed off to fight World War II.

1968: Diahann Carroll stars in the sitcom *Julia,* about a widowed single mother struggling to balance home life and work as a nurse; she's one of TV's first black lead characters.

1970: *Mary Tyler Moore* brings us television's first unapologetically single, childless, working woman over thirty and puts her quite realistically in an otherwise all-male newsroom.

1980: The movie *9 to 5* chronicles three beleaguered secretaries' united revenge on their chauvinist boss, complete with rat poison and kidnapping.

1981: *Cagney & Lacey* team up to solve crimes on TV, no men needed. Although it had taken years to sell network executives on the concept, it went on to become a huge hit.

1988: *Murphy Brown* hits the airwaves, showing us that women could work well side by side, thank you, and could even teach one another a lesson or two.

1988: *Working Girl* glorifies a Staten Island secretary who uses her bitchy boss's sick leave to get the credit she deserves — and to steal the boss's job and beau while she's at it.

2005: *Grey's Anatomy* gives us a feminist's dream world: a surgical staff stuffed with empowered, independent, driven female doctors.

2006: *The Devil Wears Prada* brings a tyrannical female boss to the screen in the form of fashion editor Miranda Priestly, played by Meryl Streep, but shows the emotional toll of stepping on underlings (in a rare female-dominated industry) to get to the top.

2006: *30 Rock* brings us Liz Lemon, a heroine torn between personal and professional life (professional always wins), who works just fine with female star Jenna Maroney but can't seem to find many decent female comedy writers to fill out her staff.

THE REAL PROBLEM: PATRIARCHY STILL KICKS US IN THE VAG

Women have not yet achieved true equality in the workplace, despite decades of great strides. A group of women spent a decade suing one of the country's largest employers, Walmart, accusing the chain of paying them lower wages and giving them fewer promotions than their male counterparts, only to lose the case in 2011. And problems like these persist despite women surpassing men in college enrollment: a 2011 White House report showed that women still make less money on average than men and are more likely to live in poverty. We lose on the home front too. Though more men than women were unemployed thanks to the so-called man-cession — male-dominated fields such as construction and manufacturing suffered more than other industries in the recent economic downturn — women still ended up below the poverty line more often than men. Why? We get the kids, so there are far more single moms holding down the fort than single dads (according to the Population Reference Bureau, there were 19.6 million single-mom households in 2009, a statistic that is cited as a major factor in child poverty as well), and yet we're still making less than men, perhaps thanks to lingering beliefs that men are breadwinners who must support families.

Granted, our American culture is to blame for that too, refusing to acknowledge men's role in parenting. While most of Europe guarantees at least some paid paternity leave, the United States does not guarantee any. Meanwhile, American women are goaded by the media to strive to have it all. And many women are burning themselves out and beating themselves up for not being able to run perfect households, raise perfect children, be perfect wives and lovers, and dominate at work while also remaining healthy, sexy, and vibrant. That would be possible only if we could bend the space-time continuum, ladies, at least until workplaces get more flexible and men are expected to take on more responsibility at home.

Problems start in our gender-specific upbringings as well. Girls are discouraged from pursuing science and math, which means that far fewer researchers and computer programmers, employees who are in particular demand these days, are female. And if you think girls' lack of skills in some fields is due to "brain differences," think again: a 2008 National Science Foundation study found girls performed as well as boys on standardized math tests; 2010's *Pink Brain, Blue Brain*, by neuroscientist Lise Eliot (a girl who does science!), shows there are few significant differences between male and female brains. "What I found, after an exhaustive search, was surprisingly little solid evidence of sex differences in children's brains," Eliot writes in the introduction to that book.

Those studies that claim to show differences don't take into account that brains change over time with every new input they receive — culture and nature can't be separated when it comes to brain research. The differences come in the way children are raised according to gender. Women are still often perceived as lacking gravitas — a problem that could be on the perceiver's side as well as the perceived's, but it's a reality we must face. And a majority of women (77 percent of those surveyed by the Center for Work-Life Policy) believe the corporate world is a meritocracy, while most men (83 percent) see it as a matter of networking. Alas, the guys are the ones who are right there. Sorry, ladies, the authors were raised as overachievers too, so we wish it were that way. It's just not.

From business (the United States had eighteen female Fortune 500 CEOs as of this writing) to NASCAR driving (yay, Danica Patrick!), cooking to comedy (yay, Melissa McCarthy!), government to finance (yay, Elizabeth Warren!), women are making inroads, but we're far from equal. In 2011, only two of *Forbes*'s Top 20 Billionaires were women (The Walmart family's Christy and Alice Walton, of all people).

THE SOLUTION: START VIEWING OTHER WOMEN AS YOUR GREATEST ALLIES

While our feminist foremothers of the 1960s envisioned women standing united to rise to equal power with men, the reality, as more and more women have entered the workplace, has been women often at odds with their female coworkers. The vision represented by the 1980 movie *9 to 5* — of female secretaries banding together to revolt against "sexist, egotistical, lying, hypocritical bigot" bosses — has hardly come to pass.

That doesn't mean we can't get there. For starters, why not seek out a female role model? You'll both benefit from the relationship: she from the relief of having another woman on her side, you from her wealth of experience in getting ahead in a sexist world. If you're in a position to be that female role model, why not seek out some younger women to mentor? You'll be helping womankind and boosting your own ego. There's nothing more fun than having starry-eyed fans who want to be just like you. Plus, if you wait five or ten years, they'll be in positions to help you out. You'll have a whole secret army of your protégées stationed across your industry, ready to do your bidding while you kick back and relax. Sure, you can mentor men too — and don't forget to seek out your own male mentor if that's who's dominating the top ranks — but the women will appreciate it more. "Mentoring makes a huge difference from both sides," Mooney says. "The woman who's the mentor might feel less threatened if she's giving advice. And to the woman being mentored, it gives more of the feeling that there's space for everyone."

The Power of Positive Role Models

Growing up in poverty in rural Mississippi during the 1960s, one young black woman never lost her spirit. Despite enduring racism in the world at large and abuse at home, Oprah Winfrey knew things were going to change for her. She knew this because of *Mary Tyler Moore.*

When the sitcom first hit the airwaves, in 1970, no one had ever seen a character like Mary Richards. She was an independent, career-driven woman in her thirties determined to make it in broadcasting. And she was single! The program redefined how women were portrayed on television. And in sweet-but-feisty Mary, a feminist icon was born. An icon who inspired millions, and not just single white midwestern women in their thirties like her; because of Mary, that young woman from Mississippi became one of the most influential women in the world. *Mary Tyler Moore* "was a light in my life, and Mary was a trailblazer for my generation," Winfrey has said.

Witness the power of a positive role model.

Role models set standards the next generation follows and seeks to raise. We women wouldn't be where we are today without the feminist icons who fought for and inspired us. We owe our right to vote to Elizabeth Cady Stanton. Sojourner Truth spoke up for all women when the abolitionist delivered her groundbreaking speech "Ain't I a Woman?" Betty Friedan gave us one of the most important feminist wake-up calls with *The Feminine Mystique,* helping women to break out of their happy-homemaker bonds — and she cofounded the National Organization for Women. Virginia Woolf and Dorothy Parker were among the first to give voice to the emotional depth and biting wit of women during times of extreme sexism. New York congresswoman Shirley Chisholm paved the way for Hillary Rodham Clinton and every other female presidential hopeful. (In 1968, Chisholm became the nation's first black congresswoman, and in 1972 she became the first major-party black presidential contender.) And Gloria Steinem made fighting for gender justice chic to generations of women. These and countless other icons were our mothers' and grandmothers' feminist role models. They planted the seeds for what's become a blooming revolution that advances and changes with every move we make.

Questions to Consider in the Workplace

1. If you're frustrated by your female boss, do you have legitimate reasons for being so?
2. Do you judge female coworkers on superficial measures such as looks or fashion? How can you move past that?
3. Be honest: Do you fight other women for power in your office? Are you vying to be "most favorite lady" in your workplace? What can you do to stop targeting other women and start working on your own career instead?
4. What one thing can you do to combat sexism in your office or your industry?
5. Do you prefer working for a male boss? If so, why? No, really — why?
6. Which younger women at your office or in your industry can you offer to mentor?
7. What networking opportunities can you seek?

Sexy Feminist Action Plan

1. Choose a female professional role model — the big, famous kind — and read up on her life, work, and philosophy to find inspiration for your own career path.
2. Look for mentoring opportunities, whether you take younger female coworkers under your wing or find a group that matches professional women with girls who need your help. Many industries have organizations dedicated to boosting fledgling female careers.

3. Stop resisting female bosses. If you have one, take her out to lunch and ask her about her career path. You might learn something, and you'll win some points. Everyone loves someone who's interested in her.

4. Go out of your way to foster a relationship with your female peers as well. They're the ones most likely to inspire competitive urges in you, so the more you like them, the better.

5. Agitate for equal representation for women at the executive table and for flexible family-leave policies, whether or not any of this will benefit you directly. A workplace that has these features is more welcoming to women as a group.

6. Ask for a raise when you deserve it. Every time this happens, at least one more woman — you! — gets closer to equal pay.

EIGHT

BE A SEXY FEMINIST, NOT A SLUT-SHAMING ONE

WE ALL KNOW THE virgin/whore dichotomy is evil, but the sexy/slutty divide seems to be another story. Otherwise-liberated women can fall into the trap of desperately trying to be sexy while cattily labeling others as slutty. So what is sexy? What is slutty? And can the distinction ever be feminist?

The way we see it, the distinction between sexy and slutty *could* be feminist if *sexy* is defined as anything that makes you feel sensuous, beautiful, and in control of your own sexuality, and *slutty* is defined as straining to please the male gaze — a gaze that is difficult, if not impossible, to satisfy, given its culturally reinforced general preference for virginal beings who are somehow also porn stars in the bedroom. Sexy has nothing to do with how many partners you've had or will have or wish to have, and everything to do with the message you're sending the world — through what you wear, how you act, what you say, and your intentions behind all three.

You could dress modestly because male figures demand it of you or because society tells you that if you don't you're "asking for it." Or you could dress modestly because you're most comfortable that way or because you don't feel the need to make your clothes a form of entertainment for every man who sees you. You could dress provocatively to beg for male attention and adulation using your most superficial qualities. Or you could dress provocatively because you want to express your sexuality or because you want to assert women's right to wear whatever we damn well please.

This, ladies, is exactly why the movement known as sex-positive feminism is so confusing. Is your desire to assert your sexuality manifested in a stretchy micro-mini worn without panties (much to your discomfort) that pleases your overbearing boyfriend? Or is it in the sumptuous satin bra and panties you wear with your favorite fishnets that make you *and* your lover wild with passion? Hint: The fishnets, in this case, are feminist. The Lycra mini could be too, if that's what *you* prefer. It's a matter of motive, and a motive only you can provide.

Sexy Feminist: Christina Aguilera

There is something to be said for evolving from a petulant teenager to an outspoken advocate for women's empowerment. Forget whether her teenybopper writhing to "Genie in a Bottle" or her assless chaps in the "Dirrty" video were feminist or not. The Mouseketeer turned powerhouse singer turned *Voice* judge models what it means to be a pop star in charge of her own artistry and destiny.

The world met Christina Aguilera in that teen-pop-saturated year of 1999. The former *All-New Mickey Mouse Club* kid stood out among the flaxen-haired, dimple-cheeked masses because of her voice. It was bigger, stronger, and more multidimensional than anything we'd heard since Mariah Carey. So we listened. And what she gave us, even from the earliest days of her career, were girl anthems about empowerment, individualism, and standing up for yourself. "Fighter," "What a Girl Wants," and "Can't Hold Us Down" championed a woman's right to call the shots and reject the double standards set forth by sexism and patriarchy. Those are some lyrics we're happy to have stuck in our heads to a catchy tune — and, even better, to have stuck in the heads of young girls around the globe.

In Christina's world, women are never reduced to pining for a man or cowering from his abuse. They're loudmouthed, opinion-ated bitches (a title she owns, Tina Fey–style) who get what they want when they want it. It's a ballsy message Madonna could get behind. She also has a softer side: her song "Beautiful" is a pow-erful celebration of individuality and difference, with a video fea-turing young people of all genders, sexual orientations, and back-grounds proclaiming their common beauty. No matter how you dress up the package, her message is one of the more feminist in popular music today.

Of course, the packaging of Christina Aguilera has always been part of the discussion surrounding her — often the loudest part. Pop star as fetish object is nothing new, but most young performers are either too naïve to reject the image forced on them by an industry still run and ruled by men or so eager to excel that they go too far (see Britney Spears). But as soon as Christina was old enough to understand her sexuality, she owned it. Sometimes that meant going a little too far, and these actions weren't without consequence; little girls everywhere wanted to wear the belly shirts and spandex she popularized during her early reign.

Aguilera has often talked about the Catch-22 of being a female performer who's pressured to showcase her physical attributes at the same time she's criticized for doing so. "Sexuality will always be a part of the way I express myself artistically. I don't think a woman should be afraid of her sexuality," she told *Cosmopolitan* in 2006. "It's not a bad thing for a woman to feel confident and show her body in a way that's right for her." The lesson: Giving in to a short-shorts trend or stuffing our bras at some point in our lives doesn't mean we can't evolve into self-aware feminists. As humans, we experiment and explore the extremes of ourselves to see where we feel most at home within our bodies. Aguilera simply did it in the public eye.

So as Aguilera evolved, she may have made mistakes — and when we say mistakes, we mean those assless chaps from the "Dirrty" video. But many a young woman has a pair of assless chaps, metaphorically speaking, in her past. Learning from it is what matters.

IS SEXY FEMINIST?

No one can argue that women's sexual expression, pleasure, and satisfaction isn't of utmost feminist importance. Hell, most young men, feminist or not, would likely support this view. Women's right to have a good time in the bedroom was one of the first feminist tenets to be embraced across both genders — sex is just more fun for both parties when women have a good time too. In fact, embracing female pleasure is what draws a lot of newcomers to the movement. But this doesn't go over so well with every activist. Writer Amanda Hess has argued that bringing sex positivity into the equation is, essentially, the activist equivalent of our aforementioned pantyless micro-mini — that it's a way of making feminism more fun, palatable, and, yes, sexy for the masses. But she's not too thrilled about that. "I think it's condescending to the feminist movement that we have to bring orgasms in to be taken seriously," she wrote on the *Washington City Paper*'s blog *The Sexist*.

And, of course, there's Ariel Levy's *Female Chauvinist Pigs* argument: that young women have internalized male standards of sexiness and used them to get attention, *Girls Gone Wild*–style, while calling it empowering. As she explained in a 2006 interview with the *Guardian*: "The whole argument that women are choosing this path themselves, and that that makes it OK, doesn't particularly make sense to me . . . I mean, I suppose it is a tiny nugget of progress, but it's like we have taken the cage away from women and none of us is trying to escape, we're just behaving exactly as we think men want us to." *New York Times* columnist Maureen Dowd, author of the book *Are Men Necessary?*, questioned this male-oriented approach to sex positivity in a 2005 piece: "Before it curdled into a collection of stereotypes, feminism had fleetingly held out a promise that there would be some precincts of womanly life that were not all about men. But it never quite materialized. It took only a few decades to create a brazen new world where the highest ideal is to acknowledge your inner slut. I am woman; see me strip."

Even the womanizing rogue Hank Moody, the character played by David Duchovny on Showtime's *Californication*, feels that boundaries are in order: "Do we think the ladies have gone too far with the sex-positive feminism?" he said in a 2009 episode. "I mean, I know they're all down with the pornography and the shaved pudenda and whatnot, but do we really think this is the path to liberation?"

Well, Hank, when you put it that way . . . no.

THE DAMAGE OF BEING TOO SEXY

There seems to be no middle ground between embracing one's inner porn star and slut-shaming the women who find themselves pressured or lured into sex-related work because they have few other options. Take the example of Melissa Petro, who became known in September 2010 as the "Hooker Teacher" after the *New York Post* "broke" the story that the South Bronx elementary school teacher used to be a prostitute and a stripper. Of course, Petro had actually broken the story herself by writing a *Huffington Post* editorial criticizing the censoring of Craigslist's adult-services section, acknowledging her past, without apology, since it was relevant to the subject. Granted, perhaps she was naïve to think word wouldn't get back to the school or that it wouldn't cause an uproar. It did, naturally, and she was fired. But worse, the media subsequently eviscerated her: there was the handy "hooker teacher" handle, which made it sound like she was holding down both jobs at the same time when in fact she'd given up sex work years earlier, gotten two master's degrees, and become a teacher while writing on the side. "Bronx Art Teacher Melissa Petro Blabs About Exploits as Stripper, Hooker," another headline said, as if writing a reasoned editorial from a specific perspective was equivalent to locker-room bragging. Worst of all, Petro said she felt her feminist credentials were being questioned, even by some female writers. We'd be more worried if she didn't call herself a feminist. Could anyone know the pitfalls of womanhood better than a woman who grew up poor, did what she felt was necessary to make ends meet, and then pulled herself up by educating herself? Sex work isn't a feminist act. But a former (or current) sex worker can be a feminist.

"As an advocate, I had long ago realized the media generally treats current and former sex workers in one of two ways: We are portrayed as victims, looked down upon and felt sorry for, too stupid to realize our own victimization; or else we are made out to be villains — dirty, cheap, and willing to do anything to satisfy our greed," Petro wrote on Salon.com. "For years, I'd fought these gross stereotypes. Now I found myself on the receiving end of it."

Perhaps we'll all be better off if we stopped blaming the sex workers themselves and instead critiqued how the same dynamics of their industry are embedded in our everyday lives: female submission to male desire, and degrading and violent behavior against women. While we sneer at prostitutes and porn stars, many of us will go well beyond our own boundaries in our desperation to please a man. No one should have to reenact porn to have a good sex life. Unless, of course, she wants to.

It is confusing business, mixing politics and sex, and not just in an Anthony Weiner way. What's so wrong, some feminists ask, with enjoying, or even participating in, porn and stripping? Others say that what's wrong is obvious: Sex work, by its nature, with mostly male bosses and customers and mostly female workers, is coercive. Much of porn relies on playing out extreme versions of male-centric fantasies about dominating and degrading sexual conquests. Studies have, indeed, found real links between porn and sexual violence. In a perfect world of equality, stripping and pornography might be just another way to enjoy human sexuality. Few fret, for instance, about male strippers or male porn stars. That's because as the world currently stands, women lose big in the sex industry.

As a result, in the completely understandable feminist fight against pornography in the 1970s, sex was often vilified to the point that some feminist groups promoted lesbian separatism as a solution. In fact, radical '70s group the Furies suggested relating only to "women who cut their ties to male privilege," theorizing that "as long as women still benefit from heterosexuality, receive its privileges and security, they will at some point have to betray their sisters, especially lesbian sisters who do not receive those benefits." Historian Lillian Faderman advocated the practice as a way for gay women to "bring their ideals about integrity, nurturing the needy, self-determination, and equality of labor and rewards into all aspects of institution building and economics." For the record, this worked for many women coming of age in the '70s: some all-lesbian communities, such as Florida's Pagoda — since relocated to Alabama and renamed Alapine — still exist today. Resident Winnie Adams, now a senior citizen, told the *New York Times*, "To me, this is the real world. And it's a very peaceful world. I don't hear anything except the leaves falling. I get up in the morning, I go out on my front deck and I dance and I say, 'It's another glorious day on the mountain.' Men are violent. The minute a man walks in the dynamics change immediately, so I choose not to be around those dynamics."

Other radical activists equated porn directly with violence, as when writer Robin Morgan declared, "Pornography is the theory, and rape is the practice." Naturally, there has been a backlash to this backlash, with a new generation of feminists in the 1980s, '90s, and beyond, including us, arguing that promoting women's sexuality should be central to the feminist cause. Sex workers' rights advocates and BDSM practitioners, as well as feminists who prioritized free speech and sexual freedom, joined the chorus in what became known as the sex-positive movement. But many of the older activists aren't buying it. Feminist author Diana Russell, who wrote the 1993 book *Against Pornography*, says, "I am opposed to the concept of 'sex positive' because a lot of sex isn't positive, it's abusive. What's more, a lot of abusive sex is invisibalized by the term."

The Real Life of Sex Workers: How Pretty Woman *Gets It All Wrong*

A Q&A with Melissa Broudo, staff attorney for the Sex Workers Project at the Urban Justice Center:

How does it hurt sex workers for us to blame and shame such women through media coverage?

Unfortunately, sex workers are often portrayed in the media as one-dimensional "characters," in articles, photographs, and other coverage that seek to label those in the industry as either "victim" or "whore." Such simplistic one-dimensional coverage perpetuates common misconceptions of sex workers, allowing a narrative to be created in popular discourse. These two distinct narratives have been created because they are easily palatable to the general public, but the effect undermines and minimizes the great spectrum of experiences and realities of all individuals who engage in transactional sex. Further, the coverage of sex workers in the media is almost always female-gendered — hiding the existence and realities of men, transgender women, and transgender men in the industry and perpetuating this notion of the female victim/whore.

How does it hurt sex workers to also sometimes glamorize what they do, as in movies like *Pretty Woman*?

Images of glamour associated with sex work are not unilaterally negative. However, certain images that perpetuate the myth that so-called high-class escorts or exotic dancers make very large sums of money and live glamorous lives can be detrimental because it trivializes the nature of the work. First of all, exotic dancers must pay out a large percentage of their tips to management and others in the clubs. Second, escorting and other forms of sex work are difficult and involve many skills. The image of glamour without further substance can demean the fact that sex work is real work. The movie *Pretty Woman*, for example, was incredibly negative in that its central message was that if a sex worker is lucky enough, she could be rescued by a wealthy and glamorous client who will get her out of the industry. This is highly problematic in its messaging on many levels, specifically its antifeminist and anti-sex-work sentiments.

What is the biggest danger sex workers face today?

Sex workers face numerous dangers, including violence from clients, violence by police, arrest/incarceration, mental and physical illness resulting from stigmatization and marginalization, and other occupational hazards generally associated with sex work. Undoubtedly the biggest danger is violence, although it is critical to look at the root of this violence. Criminalization of prostitution and the general social stigmatization of those in the sex industry allows and perpetuates violence against workers in numerous ways. One, it allows violent individuals to perceive sex workers as disposable and easy to attack without punishment (which has unfortunately proven true, as many serial killers have murdered numerous women in the industry for years before getting caught); two, it limits workers' ability to obtain police or other institutional support prior to or after an attack; three, it allows police violence, intimidation, or sexual assault to occur; and four, it furthers the marginalization and isolation of those in the industry, separating many workers from support and safety systems.

What would you suggest as a solution to the problems facing sex workers today?

I would suggest that prostitution between consenting adults be decriminalized. The criminalization of consensual adult prostitution is incredibly harmful to sex workers and victims of trafficking because it pushes the work further underground, places individuals in riskier situations than if the work were allowed to be open, and forces individuals to amass a criminal record preventing them from moving forward with their lives if they so choose. Criminalization does not solve any of the "problems" that many people quite erroneously associate with the sex industry, such as trafficking, violence, or discrimination against women. Rather, it furthers harmful and coercive conditions by forcing people to live in silence and preventing sex workers from accessing police assistance in cases of violence or trafficking. Criminalization does not help anyone — not survivors of trafficking, not voluntary workers, and not others who become enmeshed in the criminal system as a result (clients or their partners). Rather, a system that allowed people to take ownership of their bodies and rights without constant fear of arrest and violence would create a safer and more empowering way for people to work.

THE UPSIDE OF SEX POSITIVITY

First of all, we love sex, and it doesn't seem like a part of life most of us are willing to give up anytime soon, even in the name of our feminism. And arguing against pornography and stripping can easily lead to further victimizing women as beings who can't possibly take care of themselves in sexual situations and as people who don't deserve the right to free expression. That glorifies male agency once again. The traditional view that sex is inherently antifeminist ends up mirroring the most conservative, anti-woman kind of "morality." And harshly judging sex work can lead to judging the predominantly female sex workers, who generally experience enough oppression without us piling on. As Gayle Rubin, an early pro-sex feminist, argued: "A good deal of current feminist literature attributes the oppression of women to graphic representations of sex, prostitution, sex education, sadomasochism, male homosexuality, and transsexualism. Whatever happened to [blaming] the family, religion, education, child-rearing practices, the media, the state, psychiatry, job discrimination, and unequal pay?"

Not to mention that pornography isn't by its nature inherently sexist. More and more female-targeted porn is being made, much of it by female filmmakers, and an increasing number of women are watching it unabashedly. We do it for the same reasons as men — to get turned on, to get off, to live out fantasy scenarios vicariously, even to learn about sex. Some vagina activists — yes, that's a thing — even recommend watching some just to see what other women's lady parts look like and to learn to appreciate your own, though we'd caution that many porn actresses have, let's say, highly stylized versions of the standard equipment. Women should be allowed to like sex, porn, casual sex, and being kinky just as much as men do. They might not want to do these things, but they should be options. In fact, feminism can't be considered a success until that's accomplished. Nothing promotes the "good girl" ideal more than making it the only feminist option, on top of all of its other soul-crushing baggage.

We should be able to love our bodies and show them off however we want. We should feel good about ourselves and sexy in our own skin, and we should be able to flaunt it without being slut-shamed or blamed for "asking for it." Our sexuality is powerful, and we should have the chance to revel in that, not be forced to tamp it down for fear of being unfeminist. Sex is fun, healthy, intimate, and a God-given right. We should have the freedom to exercise that right as much as men.

That doesn't mean we *must* immediately embark on a tour

of strange men's beds to further the cause of feminism. (Though if you want to, we're not judging. Just make sure you use protection.) Perhaps the more straightforward, and less exhausting, way to further women's sexual liberation is to educate yourself about sex beyond the basic mechanics and to talk about it intelligently with others. Many classy sex-toy stores, which tend to be female-friendly, offer classes in everything from orgasms to erotic massage to how to use BDSM restraints. While we'd never tell you to ignore the negative side of sex — we'll say it again, be careful out there! — we also think sex is pretty cool. Get a vibrator. Get fun condoms. Read erotica. There are some wonderfully literary collections for women these days. We're fans of the several anthologies edited by Rachel Kramer Bussel. Read smart writing about sex. Nerve.com is great, sex columnist Dan Savage is great, and many other intelligent people are writing about sex. Choose your partners wisely, for whatever kind of relationship is best for you now.

THE DOWNSIDE OF SEX POSITIVITY

Of course, as wonderful as individual men can be, patriarchy can still screw with the best feminist intentions. This is when we see how lesbian separatism could be tempting. It sure would cut down on, if not eliminate, some of this confusion. For starters, we can't say all porn is good for women. Most of it, currently, is not, for women in front of the camera or women in general. We can't call stripping a feminist act if the predominantly male crowds watching don't see it that way. As onetime stripper Sarah Katherine Lewis wrote in a piece for Alternet.com, "The performances I gave didn't change anyone's ideas about women. On the contrary, I was in the business of reinforcing the same old sexist misinformation you can see in any issue of *Hustler* or *Girls Gone Wild* DVD. I wasn't 'owning' or 'subverting' anything other than my own working-class status. Bending over to Warrant's 'Cherry Pie' didn't make me a better feminist. It just made me a feminist who could afford her own rent." We're all for making feminism sexy, but it's fair to also heed Maureen Dowd's warning about "giving intellectual pretensions to a world where the highest ideal is to acknowledge your inner slut."

The sexual arena allows men to interfere in a particularly insidious way with feminist messaging, because men so often are women's partners in the act. And that's exactly where things have gotten messy now, with male-dominated corporations co-opting the concepts of supposedly empowered female sexuality. We have an authentic need to express our desires, to show off our bodies, maybe even to call ourselves sluts. But it's far from feminism when advertisements package our desires and sell them back to us as products. Think the girl power of the Spice Girls and the Pussycat Dolls, the empowerment talk that sells stripping classes. You do see the difference between the frankly sexual lyrics of, say, early Liz Phair and the fluff of the Pussycat Dolls, or between an orgasm class at progressive sex-toy store Babeland and an amateur night at a seedy strip club, right? Therein lies the difference between women's sexual agency and self-objectification. It's all in how the men figure into the equation. We don't like it either, but it's true. We're not saying we should be out to make men miserable or that we should avoid ever pleasing any male creatures with any aspects of our sexuality. We're saying that we can't make everything *just* about them.

That said, we can't quite afford to be, well, sex negative in this day and age, can we? To deny that women's sexuality is an important feminist issue is to allow patriarchal society to keep telling us what we're supposed to want and need. The trick is balancing that agenda. Society must give women the choices they deserve, which is, after all, the entire point of feminism. But women must give up the insidious urge to call anything sexual feminist in the name of sex positivity. There's a line in the 2011 romantic comedy *Crazy, Stupid, Love* when a ladies' man (Ryan Gosling) informs his protégé-in-cool (Steve Carell), "The war between the sexes is over. We won the second women started doing pole dancing for exercise." Let's embrace our sexuality without giving guys like him that particular pleasure, shall we?

Sex-Positive Feminist Icons

Madonna: Duh.

Susie Bright: Well-known erotica writer and essayist on sex; author of the inspiring — and best-selling — *Full Exposure: Opening Up to Your Sexual Creativity and Erotic Expression* and *Sexual State of the Union*

Betty Dodson: Sex educator, author, and artist widely credited for starting the sex-positive movement for women with her erotic art in the late '60s; her 1974 book *Sex for One* sold more than a million copies and sparked a masturbation movement, complete with group-masturbation workshops.

Shere Hite: Sex researcher who expanded on the pioneering work of Alfred Kinsey and Masters and Johnson with a focus on female sexuality

Eve Ensler: Pioneering playwright who helped erase women's shame about their bodies, sexuality, and femalehood with the legendary *Vagina Monologues*

Joani Blank: Founder of the country's first woman-centered sex shop, Good Vibrations, in 1977 in San Francisco

Questions to Ask Yourself About Your Sex Positivity

1. Do you have strong feelings on what's sexy versus what's slutty? Where might those feelings be coming from?

2. What outer expression of your sexuality makes you feel empowered?

3. When in your life have you strained to please a man sexually even when it felt uncomfortable and unsexy to you?

4. How do you feel about pornography?

5. How do you feel about female sex workers — strippers, porn stars, and prostitutes? Do they conjure sympathy or scorn? Why?

Sexy Feminist Action Plan: Embrace Your Inner Sex-Positive Goddess

1. Read the work of sex workers turned writers such as Carol Queen, Tristan Taormino, and Annie Sprinkle to understand their specific, informed perspectives on the industry.

2. Check out the recommendations of Toronto-based sex shop Good for Her's annual Feminist Porn Awards (http://www.goodforher.com/feminist_porn_awards).

3. Fight sex trafficking through groups such as Standing Against Global Exploitation, the Protection Project, the Coalition Against Trafficking in Women, Captive Daughters, and the Polaris Project.

4. Read the work of Robin Morgan and Catharine MacKinnon to understand the roots of anti-pornography feminism, and Ariel Levy's *Female Chauvinist Pigs* for a nuanced modern argument against female self-objectification and "raunch culture."

5. See chapter 2, "Our Poor Vaginas," to learn to love your lady parts more.

NINE

FLIRTING AND DATING: *THE RULES, THE GAME,* AND REAL LIFE

WE HAVE FOLLOWED *The Rules* now for fifteen years. The best-selling dating guide and pervasive '90s phenomenon offered up "time-tested secrets for capturing the heart of Mr. Right" from authors Ellen Fein and Sherrie Schneider. In other words, it injected into our culture a barrage of outdated, manipulative ways for heterosexual women to trick the wrong men into falling for them by using tenets of Psychology 101: Don't talk to a man first. Don't meet him halfway or go dutch on a date. Don't call him, and rarely return his calls. Don't accept a Saturday-night date after Wednesday. Always end the date first. Don't see him more than once or twice a week. No more than casual kissing on the first date. Let him take the lead.

The Rules were like the *Fight Club* for women in the '90s: There's even a Rule that tells you to do the Rules even when people tell you not to. And another that tells you not to discuss the Rules with your therapist. Maybe because he or she would tell you they were bullshit left over from 1960?

The Rules got its comeuppance a decade later thanks to *The Game*. What started as a fascinating sociological study — author Neil Strauss documenting the subculture of guys bonding over trying (and, mostly, failing) to be pickup artists — ended up playing out in pop culture as more of a how-to for dudes to trick women into bed, just as women were tricking men into weddings with *The Rules*. Thank you, *The Game*, for making *peacocking* and *negging* part of our informed dating vocabulary. (That's dressing snazzy enough to get attention, and insulting a woman so she feels the need to prove herself to you, respectively.)

One imagines these days that *The Rules* and *The Game* have been passed down from older siblings to younger ones, thus taking on the guise of ancient wisdom. And that their ideas are so ingrained in our collective unconscious that young women and young men are coming at each other in bars and restaurants to perform preordained scripts on their first dates without even realizing it. He peacocks. She lets him pay. He negs. She pecks his cheek good night by 8:00. He calls three days later, only to tell her he didn't like her dress much anyway. She doesn't return his call.

Three more days later, he calls again to tell her he hates her hair but he wants her to know he is wearing a jaunty hat. She picks up the third time he calls, but it's Thursday, so she won't go out with him until two Saturday nights from then. When they see each other again, it's been a month since their first date. They barely recognize each other when he picks her up.

This thing never had a chance. They both start over with different partners they meet the next weekend.

THE RULES DON'T WORK; HONESTY DOES

We may have gotten lower phone bills out of following the Rules, but we also got a lot of feminist guilt. For if the book was criticized for anything, it was for sending straight women back to the time before the sexual revolution. Sure, the Rules put us in charge and put us on a pedestal. But they negated any sense we had of agency and prerogative in choosing potential mates. They reinforced gender stereotypes. They underscored the "good girl" standards against which so many feminists have fought for so long. They also happened to stop the freethinking and the personal sense of control that comes from making your own decisions. Make no mistake, ladies, this kind of thing does not put you in charge — it puts the women who wrote *The Rules* in charge. If that's not enough to turn you against the Rules, consider this: It also stops authentic love from blooming. The Rules might work — briefly — if you're looking to trap a man, any man, at all costs. But ask any happy couples you know, and you're likely to hear about how their connection was so right, they forgot all the stuff they were supposed to do. They went ahead and called each other a day, or even mere hours, after the first date. They slept together on the second date. They went out on Saturday *even though he asked on Thursday.*

Both of us settled with our soul mates by completely ignoring the Rules — not that we weren't sucked into them at various points in our dating lives. Heather met the man who's now her husband when she was nineteen. They spent years apart, often separated by thousands of miles, dating other people, establishing careers, and growing up. They spent some years together successfully; others not so successfully. They eventually reunited ten years after their first meeting and settled down, each with the person who had made sense all along.

Jennifer met her longtime boyfriend online, and though both she and Jesse were jaded New Yorkers who, between the two of them, had been on approximately a million unproductive dates, they forgot every boundary they had by the end of their first date. Jennifer told him she could stay for only one drink because she had to get home to blog *Grey's Anatomy,* which was both true and strategic — if she liked him, she figured, she'd seem busy and important and alluringly indifferent; if she didn't, she'd get out quick. She was there for three hours, which meant staying up until four in the morning to blog *Grey's Anatomy.* He, in turn, lost all sense of propriety and e-mailed her as soon as he got home from their date to ask for another one. She answered at 4:01 A.M., as soon as she was done blogging. They've now been together for two years, Rules be damned.

As Naomi Wolf wrote in *The Beauty Myth,* "Sadly, the signals that allow men and women to find the partners who most please them are scrambled by the sexual insecurity initiated by beauty thinking. A woman who is self-conscious can't relax to let her sensuality come into play. If she is hungry she will be tense. If she is 'done up' she will be on the alert for her reflection in his eyes. If she is ashamed of her body, its movement will be stilled. If she does not feel entitled to claim attention, she will not demand that airspace to shine in. If his field of vision has been boxed in by 'beauty' — a box continually shrinking — he simply will not see her, his real love, standing right before him." That book, incidentally, came out in 1991, five years before *The Rules*. It's as if Wolf was explicitly trying to warn us of that book's coming. Alas, many women didn't listen.

Flirting and dating are most warped by sexism when it comes to heterosexual relationships, so that's where feminist-proofing becomes the hardest. And if you want to attract a feminist man, the right feminist man, the rules are not going to do it. (Note: There are rules in gay relationships too. A lesbian labors over wearing the right thing on a date, being too forward, and counting the days until she calls. But we're going to focus on heterosexual relationships here because they are what these rules — and the sexual politics that define our male-run, male-dominated culture — were created for. Gay women have an advantage in this one case: There are no penis politics at play in their relationships.)

And yet, without the Rules, or even the billions of other sets of rules regularly spewed at us through the years by self-help books and women's magazines, how do we know how to react to the constant emotional traps of dating? Imagine life without a chorus of advisers telling you how to navigate love: You might just talk to a man whenever you felt like it. You might meet him at a mutually convenient location for your date. You might see him three times in one week. You might pour your soul out to him if he seems willing to listen.

It sounds terrifying, all this following of your own instincts and making your own decisions. If things happened to go wrong, you'd self-flagellate for months, maybe even years, worried you'd screwed up your one chance at happiness. We know, because we've each done this once or twice.

But it also sounds a lot like a dream relationship. The truth is, there is no surefire plan for finding true love. There are only elaborate systems of distraction meant to give you something to do while you wait for the right person to show up. Women spend their time following rules; men play games.

The Feminist Rules

These apply equally to heterosexual and lesbian, bisexual, and transsexual women.

1. Don't assume your date is paying, but don't feel like a traitor to feminism if he or she does.
2. Chivalry is just good manners. Feel free to reciprocate.
3. Be yourself at all costs.
4. Talk to any potential partner you feel like talking to, anytime you feel like talking to him or her, about whatever you feel like discussing.
5. End phone calls and dates when you feel like it.
6. You don't need rules to tell you when you can call or see your crush again. But if he or she is going to ask you on a date, make that person really ask you out. We notice lately

that young men, in particular, think it's okay to text *Where U at?* to someone and consider that an invitation to spend quality time together. That's not romantic. We're not even sure if it's cool for our friends to do that, much less potential partners.

7. Dump anyone who's freeloading, disrespectful, ill-mannered, inattentive, or unresponsive.

8. Speak up if you disagree with something he or she is saying. If you think your date is well intentioned but wrong, you can do this firmly but sweetly. If your date is a jerk, you can do this before dumping him or her per no. 7.

9. Follow your feelings. This does not include stalking your crush or losing all sense of normalcy; if you think you shouldn't call/e-mail/text just yet, you probably shouldn't. Tune in to your instincts the best you can. (We know it's hard. But you can do it!)

10. When it comes to getting physical, know what's right for you and stick to it. If sex too early usually comes back to hurt you later, hold off. If it doesn't bug you or you're more interested in sex than a relationship, do whatever you like (with protection, please!).

11. We're down with three of the original Rules: Don't tell him or her what to do; don't expect a lover to change or try to change him or her (no good, feminist or otherwise, is going to come from that); and don't date married people! (So not feminist.)

12. Be honest.

13. See dating as a chance to get to know other cool human be-

ings, practice your conversation skills, and learn new things. This way, you never lose.

14. Take care of yourself first.

FEMINISM AND RELATIONSHIPS DO *GO HAND IN HAND*

Here's the main problem when women get into these issues of sexuality and feminism: If you're straight, sex is the one place men get to mess with you, by definition. That is not to say you should let them *really* mess with you, but you cannot separate men from the issue the way you can when it comes to pursuing your career or fighting for political rights. Even a smart feminist woman can find herself paging through *The Rules* looking for answers after running into her ex with his young new girlfriend. A feminist who's gone on one too many bad dates can find herself letting it slide when a hot prospect scoffs about how feminists are so annoying or how hideous Hillary Clinton is or how ridiculous it is that all these female comics think they can be funny. None of us is proud of these moments later. But under the influence of loneliness and hormones, things happen.

In a strange, twisted way, *The Rules* — as well as its descendants, like *He's Just Not That Into You* — were trying to come to feminists' aid. It's good to have a system in place to temper your impulsive reactions when dopamine and oxytocin are rendering you senseless, a system that stops you from jumping at the first attractive man you see in a bar, from calling that new crush five times a day, from rushing into physically or emotionally unsafe sex, from concocting fantasies surrounding a romantic target instead of seeing him for what he is. These and many other attempts to give control to women — the dating site AdoptaGuy.com, for example, which allows women to "shop" for men they'd like to date — may be well intentioned, but they're also misguided. Putting women on a pedestal in any way by saying *they're* the only ones qualified to take control of relationships and "train" men to behave just perpetuates the idea that women must be all sweetness and light, men must be all sex drive and stupidity, and never the twain shall meet (except to have unequal, unsatisfying, disconnected sex and relationships).

Another major roadblock on the way to feminist relationship satisfaction has been the persistent question from social conservatives of whether feminism has made women happier. When they say *happier*, they mean "married with children and without (acknowledged) conflict." *Flipside of Feminism* coauthor Suzanne Venker (who wrote the book with her notoriously antifeminist mom, Phyllis Schlafly) declared in 2011, "Feminism has sabotaged women's happiness." In the widely discussed book, she and Schlafly cited the emasculation of men (which hurts women's happiness how?), the exhaustion of women (women are too tired for sex, apparently), and the reluctance of women to settle down and marry (again, this means women aren't happy?) as evidence. The truth is that feminism means choices, and choices breed discontent, because of some irritating quirk in human psychology. Does that mean our lives are worse? No; it just means we have more shit to think about. There's no doubt we're putting off marriage and kids longer, giving more time to our careers and less time to pining for love, and asking more from love than ever before. Gone are the days when women married the first men they could find just for lifelong security and baby-making. All of that is bound to have an effect on societal indicators of commitment, but that doesn't make us less happily-ever-after, just more skeptical of an erroneous concept. We'd rather be free and thinking than happy. And the veracity of happiness studies is another subject altogether. Scientists can't even figure out if wine, aspirin, and fish are good or bad for us; why should we trust researchers to measure an intangible idea like happiness?

The media is, overall, of little help. When commentators are not warning us about feminism's detrimental effects on marriage or women's ticking-time-bomb biological clocks, they're offering up some of the most offensive "solutions" to those "problems" possible. From women's magazines to *The Millionaire Matchmaker*, we hear loads of specific advice about how to attract a man, how to keep a man, how to please a man. *Matchmaker*'s Patti Stanger extols the man-snagging virtues of long hair, big boobs, and few friends (they're competition; duh), and advises demanding large gifts from suitors (jewelry preferred). *Cosmo* thinks we should "Cook dinner topless, apply a little tomato sauce to your nipple (make sure it's not too hot), and ask your man if it's spicy enough." Yeah, that's *really* from the October 2010 issue. God, how do the A-cups among us ever find love and happiness?

The problem, of course, is the fair success rate of all these approaches — *The Rules, The Game, He's Just Not That Into You, The Millionaire Matchmaker, Cosmo* — all the way back to the granddaddy of offensive advice based on traditional gender roles, *Men Are from Mars, Women Are from Venus*. (From the 1992 smash bestseller: "A woman's sense of self is defined through her feelings and the quality of her relationships." "Just as a man is fulfilled through working out the intricate details of solving a problem, a woman is fulfilled through talking about the details of her problems.") You may notice yourself nodding along to a lot of these ideas: *I do like to talk about my problems! Every guy I've dated does prefer my hair long! He does love when I put marinara sauce on my tits!* Because, well, some parts of them may be true. Human nature has a lot of annoying stuff built into it, including heterosexual men's instinctive love of "feminine" attributes (that means long hair in current culture, boobs in all cultures) and possibly of the chase, or at least a challenge, which both genders tend to love (hence, the Rules simulate a chase). Just because it's human nature doesn't mean it's best or right for modern society, though; that's why we've cut back on killing one another in the last couple thousand years.

We do not — repeat, *do not* — need to treat our potential mates as aliens with different psyches from ours, even if those people happen to have penises. As feminist psychologist Naomi Weisstein said way back in a 1969 issue of *Psychology Today*, "Except for their genitals, I don't know what immutable differences exist between men and women. Perhaps there are some other unchangeable differences; probably there are a number of irrelevant differences. But it is clear that until social expectations for men and women are equal, until we provide equal respect for both sexes, answers to this question will simply reflect our prejudices." Sexist scientists, in other words, make sexist science. Weisstein also said in the journal *Feminism and Psychology* in 1993, "Let us return to an activist, challenging, badass feminist psychology." Let us, indeed.

In fact, we're thinking "challenging, badass feminist psychology" would make a great mantra for any of us as we embark upon the often soul-crushing world of dating. It's a place where it's easiest to lose our feminism and most critical that we don't. If you're searching for Mr. Right, shouldn't he love you in all your activism, feminism, and general badassery? Shouldn't he show up when he says he will, call when he says he'll call? Shouldn't he be not just okay with your feminism but a feminist himself? Until you find that guy — yes, they exist — you should not be in a relationship. Easier said than done, we know. That's why we're talking about it now, when everyone is rational, instead of when you're depressed or horny. If you are feeling one of those things right now, sorry! We love you. You're fabulous. You don't need him, whomever you're pining for. Focus on finding the guy we just described above. Is not a bubble bath or a delicious meal or good wine or a trip to the batting cages on a spring day more worth your time than some sexist schlub? The answer is yes. *Yes.* In fact, as Pamela Haag, who wrote *Marriage Confidential,* the definitive 2011 look at modern matrimony, says: "It's about giving ourselves permission to expect better. And it's about not falling for the neo-traditional revival that would have us believe that men and women inhabit fundamentally alien worlds, or that the 'working mother' has destroyed civilization, or that we all should be trying to please men through being quiet, doing what they want, and tricking them into marrying us. Not only is that regressive, anti-feminist tripe, it's also not even good dating advice."

But does expecting better require us each to find an actually *feminist* partner? We say yes. He doesn't have to donate monthly to Planned Parenthood and lead rallies to revive the ERA. But he does have to subscribe to basic tenets such as women's right to equality, choices, and self-sufficiency. We're not sure any guy who doesn't believe in those things could be much fun on a date, much less good in bed or worth long-term commitment or gene-mixing. "We need to be willing — and brave enough — to be clear about what we expect," Haag adds.

And for us, that means an "activist, challenging, badass feminist psychology." We hope it does for you too.

Questions to Ask Yourself About Dating While Feminist

1. What rules (or Rules) do you follow? Why?
2. How do you feel about *The Rules* and *The Game,* as a feminist?
3. How have dating rules helped or hindered your love life in the past?
4. What have you done in the name of love that gave you feminist guilt?
5. Where do you turn for dating advice? Is it feminist?
6. What does your dream relationship look like?
7. How do you handle basic gender-driven dating dilemmas like who's paying, who's planning, and who's calling whom?

Sexy Feminist Dating Action Plan

1. Follow our feminist dating rules!
2. Vow to speak up for your beliefs when *anyone* — especially a romantic prospect — says something antifeminist. You can do it gently, nicely, even playfully, but do it firmly. Maybe it'll

lead to a great discussion — a lot of couples thrive on a little verbal combat. (For example, Heather and her husband. They love a good debate over who'll win the Oscars or whether Lady Gaga is feminist, among many other things.)

3. Be honest with yourself about budding relationships, and cut them off if they're not good or right for you. This is not about settling down with whoever comes along; it's about finding someone who supports you and enhances your greatness.

4. Give up on the idea of lifelong happiness, period. Sometimes you will be happy, sometimes you will not. Just worry about finding the life that's best for you, including finding the right partner for you now. That doesn't mean that love isn't out there for you; it is. It's just not *all* that's out there to make your life fulfilling. You are responsible for your own happiness; a partner merely enhances it.

5. Swear off media that tries to scare you into settling down, getting married, having kids, or anything else you don't want to do.

6. Stop buying anti-woman relationship-advice books! Just because an approach to relationships works doesn't mean you should use it. You might attract men that way, but you want to attract the right men. And it probably wouldn't last anyway.

7. Repeat after us: "Let us return to an activist, challenging, badass feminist psychology."

TEN

FEMINISM IN THE BEDROOM

H<small>E WANTS YOU TO WEAR</small> booty shorts or initiate a three-some or post amateur porn online, to be the embodiment of his schoolboy fantasies. Or maybe he wants to do it without a condom just this once — don't you trust him to be disease-free, baby? Antifeminists want you to quit bed-hopping and settle down with a nice man already. They're even sure that bed-hopping is making you, and a lot of other people, very sad, or at least less happy than the nice, chaste girls of the 1950s. Everyone was so much happier then, claim people who do surveys, not noting that such nice, chaste girls had a whole different definition of happiness! (As noted in earlier chapters: Fuck happiness studies.) Media reports want you to quit screwing around and listen to your biological clock, to fight hookup culture, to believe you are less capable of orgasms if you're smart and successful.

Feminism and heterosexual sex have often had a rocky relationship. In the days of the sexual revolution, feminist sex seemed fun to men — all braless frolicking and free love and sex without consequences, thanks to the pill. Now feminism is depicted as a buzzkill that questions media-made fantasy women, demands proper use of condoms, and makes women *think* too much. "There's this idea that feminism is bad for sex, that it's unsexy, because we insist on things like consent," says Jaclyn Friedman, the author of *What You Really Really Want: The Smart Girl's Shame-Free Guide to Sex and Safety.* "If that's unsexy, you probably have a partner who won't give you very good sex."

There's even science aimed at kicking feminism out of the bedroom: "Most women prefer to play a submissive role in the bedroom," neuroscientist Ogi Ogas told ABC News, explaining his 2011 book *A Billion Wicked Thoughts.* "We've got these primal sources of sexual arousal hard-wired in the brain. . . . It appears that in females the circuits are hooked up to be aroused by submission — usually." He added, "If you're a woman, or a man, and your preferred role is submissive, if you feel compelled to approach sex with the same gender equality as the working world, it's going to be hard to be aroused." Yes, he's trying to tell us equality is a huge boner-shrinker. The headline on that story was "Feminism as the Anti-Viagra." All most modern feminists want is satisfying sex with regular orgasms, though, and how that's anything but sexy is beyond us.

It seems downright ludicrous to say women's liberation could dampen the mood in bed for anyone but the most insecure partner. "The best way to make your sex life more egalitarian is to refuse to sleep with men who *aren't* egalitarian," *What You Really Really Want* author Friedman says. "That sounds flip, but I think there's a mentality right now that we're working in a scarcity model, that all sexuality has to be run on men's agenda. You know, 'If I want X, he's going to think I'm too demanding and go somewhere else.' That's a mass delusion. If we start en masse to stand up for our boundaries, men will have to get with the program." This is one of those areas where gay women may share some, but not all, of straight women's difficulties. Two women having sex doesn't make for a power-dynamic problem, though lesbians have grown up in the same media-saturated culture full of women who are both overly sexualized and stripped of their rights to natural desire.

Because of those and other patriarchal issues, feminism can complicate women's bedroom moods, too, if we let it. Maybe we *want* to wear booty shorts. Does that make us bad feminists? We read *Female Chauvinist Pigs*; maybe we're subconsciously objectifying ourselves. Maybe that's why we want to wear the booty shorts! Or maybe we like boring, vanilla, monogamous sex while all the sex-positive blogs are touting the joys of anal beads, bondage, polyamory, and no-strings-attached relationships. Maybe we should be making more of a statement, living our lives like promiscuous men. Are we bad feminists if we *don't?* And all this angst is without even getting to the *really* fraught feminist sex dilemmas, like BDSM and rape fantasies.

You get the point: there's almost no sex-related act that can't be somehow twisted into an antifeminist act and thus bring on massive feminist guilt. With all this tugging of our sexual psyches in so many directions, it's a wonder anyone gets laid anymore. Let's face it, women are bred these days to feed on guilt, and we've turned feminism into one more way to get our fix. Figure in sex and all of its attached moral strings, and you're in for one guilty ride. If there's one reason men still have the upper hand in straight sexual relationships, it's that we're too wrapped up in our own guilt to leave them even if we want to, and too wrapped up in our own guilt to enjoy them without commitment even if we want to.

Making Sex Safe — for Yourself and All Women

Pregnancy prevention has always been a feminist issue, for obvious reasons. As early as 1870, activists were referring to "voluntary motherhood" to underline the importance of controlling the timing of births in women's lives. The phrase *birth control* first entered the English language in 1914 and gained popularity throughout the teens and twenties, as nurse Margaret Sanger opened America's first family-planning clinic. The idea has courted controversy since its inception, given that its basic premise separated sex from the purpose of procreation. Some religions, most notably Catholicism, have expressed their displeasure with the concept, making it a fraught battle. Though it should be noted that a 2011 Guttmacher Institute study found 69 percent of religious women — and 98 percent of Catholic women! — who are sexually active use some form of birth control.

Condoms, diaphragms, and other barrier methods remain essential — the first in preventing sexually transmitted infections, the last two in offering a nonhormonal alternative to pills and shots — but the pill gets the most feminist heat. That might be because it's credited with kicking off the sexual revolution and the feminist movement in the 1960s, and thus, in many conservative eyes, it's the cause for all of our newfangled problems like casual sex, teen pregnancy, and the decline of marriage. (Never mind that it prevents unwanted children born to teens as well as adults or that unwanted marriage is no prize either.) Nonetheless, a hundred million women throughout the world are now on the pill, even as we still fight for better access and insurance coverage.

Birth control has become a part of the average woman's life, whether or not some politicians and religious leaders like it. For many modern American women, desire for a birth control prescription prompts their first visit to the gynecologist and keeps them coming back annually throughout their twenties and thirties. We get passionate about our chosen methods, proselytizing to girlfriends about the wonders of our pills, NuvaRings, patches, or Depo-Provera shots. Those of us with adequate insurance coverage take for granted our ability to not have kids when we don't want them, and to have kids when we're ready. (An issue that has gotten sticky as we've put off kids for longer, but that doesn't negate the wonders of birth control.)

Still, there are ways we can help the cause of reproductive rights for all in our everyday lives. First, we can talk about it with our friends, partners, and doctors, openly and without shame, both to further everyone's education and to erase the age-old stigma attached to a lady seeking birth control. We can fight for thorough sex education in our schools, teaching that goes beyond abstinence and gives young people straight-up facts about ways to prevent unplanned pregnancies, and for unrestricted access to birth control for the underprivileged women who need it most. That includes Plan B emergency contraception for teenagers (despite the Obama administration's restrictions on that) and safe, legal abortion access for all.

It's also imperative to do your own research when you're considering which birth control method is right for you — just because it's available, or prescribed, doesn't mean it's safe. (Class-action lawsuits against the manufacturers of Yaz and Yasmin prompted the FDA to require stronger warning labels about the danger of blood clots and highlighted the fact that these drugs we put in our bodies every day are far from benign.) Also, stay on top of what's available, and pay attention to whether your chosen method is still working for you. What worked when you were nineteen might not work when you're twenty-nine, and there may now be better options for you. Not to mention some risks on certain medications increase with age. Just one more bummer when it comes to getting older, but one that's easy to handle if you address it with your doctor.

More than anything, talking with your partner about your options is essential. Men should be included in the discussion, aware of the risks and benefits, and responsible for shouldering some of the costs if that's what you'd like. The "You're on the pill, baby, right?" comment in the heat of the moment does not count as this discussion. In fact, we dream of a day when birth control is an issue for all of us to care about, rather than just a women's issue.

In short, adequate birth control means fewer unwanted children, fewer abortions, healthier babies and mothers, lower Medicaid costs for the federal government, environmentally friendly population control, more life choices for women (and men), and more sexual freedom. Birth control boasts many ancillary benefits as well: It can decrease reproductive health problems such as fibroids and endometriosis. It can clear up acne, regulate periods, and lessen severe PMS symptoms. Some gay women go on the pill for just those reasons.

But of course, there are downsides to birth control prescriptions as well, just as there are for any drugs. They can create a false sense of security that allows you to get lax about putting a barrier between you and STIs with a new partner who hasn't been tested recently or isn't being monogamous with you. (Seriously, are condoms — cheap, effective barriers against unwanted pregnancy *and* life-threatening illnesses — not the greatest invention of modern times?) Pills, in particular, require strict adherence to a daily schedule — they're 91 to 99 percent effective, and yet how many times have you heard a surprised, newly pregnant woman say, "My birth control failed!" There are the basic health risks of new pills, like Yaz's and Yasmin's strokes and blood clots. Other far from deadly but nonetheless concerning side effects of various pills can include decreased sex drive, depression, and decreased lubrication. It's worth checking out other methods as well: intrauterine devices are more than 99 percent effective, as are vasectomies, guys!

A world without birth control would be nothing short of a negation of all of feminism's gains. (Yes, all.) Our lives would look like the domestic prisons of the 1950s or the stifling propriety of Elizabethan times — or maybe even a little like the special hell the girls on MTV's *16 and Pregnant* show us, full of deadbeat dads and dead-end futures. Just forty years ago, it was a crime in many states for unmarried people to possess birth control or information about it. In Connecticut, it was a crime for *anyone* to have it or talk about it up until the landmark Supreme Court decision *Griswold v. Connecticut.* Can you imagine? Let's not. For no more than about

$15 to $50 per month (the average cost of a copay for pills), we gain nothing less than control over our own futures. It's hard to imagine a better bargain.

Questions to Guide Your Birth Control Decisions

1. Do you need to prevent STIs or simply to protect against unwanted pregnancy? If you're in a nonmonogamous relationship or enjoying casual sex, you'll need to use condoms in addition to another method. If you're monogamous and you both have a clean bill of health from recent testing, you can rely on pills, patches, NuvaRings, IUDs, or Depo-Provera.

2. Can you remember to take a pill every day at the same time? If so, the pill is an easy option for many women and more than 99 percent effective if taken correctly. If you can't, consider the patch, which sticks to your skin and delivers hormones straight into your bloodstream.

3. Do you hate the idea of pills or patches? If you don't mind the awkwardness of getting a plastic ring up inside yourself, NuvaRing can be a worry-free and effective method.

4. Still uneasy with your options? Consider having an IUD inserted by your physician. It allows you to relax, involves fewer hormones, is reversible at any time, and is much less damaging to your reproductive system than it used to be. We can't imagine why these have fallen in popularity in recent years — they're kind of awesome.

5. Don't mind seeing your doctor every few months for a shot? Try Depo-Provera — just make sure you never miss your scheduled appointment.

6. Already messed up and had unprotected sex? You have seventy-two hours to get yourself an emergency-contraception pill (so it's a little longer than just the morning after).

7. Suffer from debilitating PMS, or just hate dealing with tampons? Ask your doctor about Seasonale or another continuous-dose pill that allows periods only every few months.

A Brief History of Birth Control

3000 B.C.: The condom is invented in Egypt.

1844: Rubber condoms — washable and reusable! — are first produced.

1873: The Comstock Laws on obscenity make all use of contraceptives illegal in the U.S.

1916: In Brooklyn, nurse Margaret Sanger opens the first family-planning clinic; it's shut down for violating a law prohibiting non-physicians from distributing birth control.

1918: Condoms become legal in the United States.

1921: Sanger founds the National Birth Control League, which educates women about ways to prevent unplanned pregnancy and will later become Planned Parenthood.

1960: The first birth control pill, Enovid, is approved by the FDA, kicking off the sexual revolution and the modern feminist movement.

1965: The Supreme Court rules in *Griswold v. Connecticut* that the U.S. Constitution protects a "right to marital privacy" that extends to the use of contraceptives, striking down a Connecticut law prohibiting them.

1992: The first hormone shot that prevents pregnancy for several months at a time, Depo-Provera, is approved.

1998: The first emergency contraception is approved.

2003: The first continuous birth control pill — the kind that reduces the number of menstrual periods — is approved by the FDA.

February 2011: Reproductive rights activists call the Republican-dominated Congress's efforts to slash Planned Parenthood and other federal family-planning funding "a war on women's health" and stage rallies throughout the country to protest; the funding survives.

December 2011: The Health and Human Services secretary publicly overruled the FDA, refusing to allow emergency contraceptives to be sold over the counter to anyone, including young teenagers.

So what *does* feminist sex look like, besides lesbian separatism? Here's our fantasy scenario: You in whatever makes you feel sexiest, feeling confident enough to try any crazy thing that crosses your dirty mind and secure enough to tell him you'd rather not fulfill his particular request tonight, if that's how you feel. The right protection to make everyone feel safe — preventing pregnancy when needed, preventing disease when not monogamous and/or not recently tested. As much sex as you desire, with as many or as few partners as you'd like, and partners of the gender or genders you prefer. Girl-on-girl make-outs only for the pleasure of those making out, not for the titillation of men who may be watching and drooling. Guilt-free, satisfying orgasms for all, however you choose to get there. Submission, domination, vibrators, oral, anal, soft, hard, and anything else you can think of. *That* is what feminist sex is made of.

Nonetheless, some specific practices have ignited debates

among feminists themselves, of course. We can't get off guilt-free! BDSM has ignited the most recent debate: A significant portion of second-wavers — namely, the same women who fought, and still fight, against porn — argue that anything that resembles sexual violence, including your basic restraint/domination, perpetuates rape culture, allows women to further internalize oppression, and ultimately hurts all women. (Some feminists have even argued that in our society, *all* sex is violent, period, as we discussed in chapter 8.) But sex-positive feminists have countered that to rule out something many women enjoy is in itself misogynistic, and they point out that dominance and submission aren't always fixed to gender roles. Meanwhile, increasing numbers of feminist bloggers and message-boarders have been coming out as, well, rather fond of being tied up. "The argument that women who enjoy BDSM are 'taught' they should be submissive in bed is insulting to me as a feminist: I'm not a little girl who needs other people to tell me what's best for me," feminist writer Jessica Wakeman told *Jezebel* in 2010. "I choose to trust the men I 'play' with." Jaclyn Friedman defends submissive tendencies this way: "I think that sexuality can be a kind of adult playground. It can be a place where we can play out things that scare us in safe ways. A lot of feminists spend all day long fighting against that, so the idea that we want a space where we can explore what that feels like feels completely natural to me."

It's hard to measure these things statistically, but put it this way: One guy we know and love tells us, "Almost every woman I've slept with, and every woman most of my friends have slept with, likes to be tied up occasionally." Explanatory theories about this abound, from an innate female desire to feel "taken" to an urge to make the bedroom the modern woman's one sanctuary where she doesn't have to do it all. Let's face it: When you're with a man you trust, getting tied up can be more relaxing than violent. He's going to let you out of the restraints and go get you a nice glass of wine once both of you have come.

Granted, taking these sorts of practices farther requires more thought and discussion. More advanced BDSM techniques — spanking, whipping, and the like — require extensive conversation with your partner before you get out the leather. (Pick a safe word and so forth.) And rape fantasies . . . well, those take submission to a whole new, and more politically charged, level. In these discussions, it's most important to remember that it's *very* unfeminist to police other women's fantasies. These fantasies are not what the women who have them want in real life; studies show that such fantasies are commonly not graphically violent. That is to say, the only part of the fantasies that is violent is the fact that the sex is forced.

Fascinatingly, researchers have traced this back to residual guilt about sexual pleasure. Nancy Friday, who documented women's desires in her 1973 book *My Secret Garden*, found rape fantasies stayed relatively consistent from that time through her 1992 update *Women on Top*. "The most popular guilt-avoiding device was the so-called rape fantasy — 'so-called' because no rape, bodily harm, or humiliation took place in the fantasy," she wrote in the update. "It simply had to be understood that what went on was against the woman's will. Saying she was 'raped' was the most expedient way of getting past the big No to sex that had been imprinted on her mind since early childhood. (Let me add that the women were emphatic that these were not suppressed wishes; I never encountered a woman who said she really wanted to be raped.)" Adds Jaclyn Friedman, who is a survivor of sexual assault: "I think rape fantasies are fine. They're really natural in a world in which rape is a public health epidemic. . . . You need to explore it with someone you trust."

Many of us, however, can feel guilty and shameful about far less complicated sexual situations than rape fantasies. No surprise, since what we've really internalized over the years is that *no* we're supposed to say whenever sexual arousal occurs. The message we get these days is more nuanced than that force-fed to women in decades past, and we're all the more confused for it. Now we're still in charge of sexual gatekeeping and still not supposed to have desires of our own, but we *are* supposed to compete with porn stars for men's sexual attention. We're supposed to always look sexually available without ever desiring sexual pleasure of our own. How patriarchy managed to trick us into this one, we'll never know. Actually, we *do* know: it's called mass media. From ads to sitcoms, we're shown silly, horny husbands who can't get enough, and wives who roll their eyes at the prospect or use it to bargain with to get chores done. Nothing inherently wrong with the chores thing, we guess, but it seems more feminist and relationship-friendly to just negotiate these things truthfully like grownups.

We're not saying real life doesn't sometimes interfere with sex lives, or desires between partners don't wax and wane over the course of a relationship. But the onus always being on the woman presents numerous feminist problems: It makes women the lame ones, the party poopers, while desexualizing us — which can make those of us with healthy sexual appetites feel like deranged nymphos. And it equates manhood with sexual desire, sending both genders into existential crises the minute the guy isn't in the mood one night. A 2011 study by psychologist Terri Fisher at Ohio State University found that men thought about food as much as they thought about sex, contrary to popular opinion, and they average just eighteen sexual thoughts per day, far fewer than the oft-quoted every-seven-seconds statistic, and not far off from the ten per day women have.

Point being, the genders are more sexually equal than we've been led to believe — and more now than ever before. There's no better time to make sex feminist.

Feminist Confessions: Playing the Fantasy Girl

He wanted me to wear short-shorts. Like Daisy Duke short-shorts, half-inch-inseam short-shorts, the kind one could purchase from the Victoria's Secret clothing collection in the mid-1990s. He gave them to me under the guise of a gift for some occasion — our one-year anniversary, perhaps — but I had not worn them outside our dorm-room walls because they were a bit (go figure) short for my comfort. I would wear them at home or in the bedroom, meaning our respective campus-housing cells, as I did not mind spicing up our nascent sex life. But I did not go anywhere (where would I go in these, anyway?) with them barely covering my ass in everyday life.

Then, suddenly, he was angry with me. Sulky, barely speaking, passive-aggressive angry. At first, he refused to tell me why, insisting I should instinctively know. Then, after some frustrating phone conversation, our first conflict in more than a year of dating, I dragged it out of him: he was mad I had not intuited his desire for me to don the short-shorts for Dillo Day, an outdoor music festival at Northwestern University. Apparently it should have been obvious that his buying me the shorts and presenting them to me in early spring meant that I was obligated, due to my undying gratitude for said shorts, to frolic in them at the pinnacle of the season.

I told him he was nuts; he told me I didn't understand his tender feelings. But I moved past it, resigned to sometimes not understanding the love of my life's every thought.

Or at least I thought I'd moved past it.

In reality, I'd have the same fight with the same man again and again, and again, from the time we met in college when I was nineteen to the time we broke up for good ten years later. The garments and desires changed — sometimes it was a thong, sometimes it was a miniskirt with no underwear, sometimes it was a dirty picture, sometimes it was a threesome. But it was always the same tiresome dance: he'd ask me to do something I didn't like, I'd express my hesitation, he'd accuse me of being cold to his advances, I'd be left to agonize over whether I should stick to my guns in the name of feminism or give in for the sake of the man I loved.

I didn't get out of the cycle until I got out of the relationship. But this constant struggle wormed its way into not only our sex life — which was otherwise, it should be noted, quite robust, and not at all vanilla — but also my self-esteem. I hadn't come to college with a wide frame of sexual reference, as the only two boys I'd loved in high school were a strict Catholic and a closeted future gay best friend. When, during my sophomore year of college, I found the man I thought I was going to marry, I wanted to make him happy. Until, it seemed, he told me *what* would make him happy. These weren't the typical things you read in women's magazines that you *don't have to do if you don't want to*. They seemed kind of, mostly, harmless. I would find myself thinking, *Why don't I want to go to the bar wearing this short skirt with no panties? What's the harm in giving my future husband this little thrill?* This line of thought soon unraveled into something more like *What's wrong with me that I don't feel comfortable doing this? Why am I so frigid and unsexy?*

I think this urge to look for what's broken in ourselves when our sex lives aren't going as planned starts, like so many neuroses, with women's magazines. When we are bombarded with "75 Naughty Sex Moves Men Crave Most" (*Cosmo,* May 2011), we think it is our duty to go through these checklists, one point at a time, and accomplish sexiness the same way we accomplish career or academic objectives, relationship or baby-raising success, and beauty or fitness goals in our idealized-superwoman times. If we do not manage to do all this, the reasoning goes, it is because we are not trying hard enough. It is a personal failing, a sign of a defect.

I did not share these struggles with anyone at the time. I wanted so badly for my friends and family to believe that my relationship was perfect, that I had pleased my man the same way I'd pulled my undergrad grade point average up to a 3.5 after dipping close to the 2 range in my freshman year — by applying my iron ambition and steel will. Meanwhile, as we were moving in together, my boyfriend was complaining I never initiated sex, and, well, he was right — I was afraid starting anything would lead to something I didn't want to do. The non-vanilla sex life devolved into a barely existent one. We decided this was a spectacular time to get engaged.

He asked, "Will you marry me?" I said, "Yes." But I couldn't parse the questions at the core of our relationship: What happens when your partner's sexual wishes irritate you? Do you give him what he wants in the name of love, as I so often did? Or do you stand up for your own feelings in the name of feminism? And it bothered me that all this bothered me: Wasn't he *supposed* to be telling me what he wanted in bed? Wasn't that what all the sex self-help books told us?

We eventually broke up for a million interrelated, complicated reasons, the buildup of ten years of sacrifices and regrets compounded by two lives pulling in opposite directions until they shattered. I never figured out the answers to those questions. At least I didn't think I did, until I noticed two curious related phenomena in subsequent relationships: One, I broke up with anyone whose tastes in the bedroom didn't blend with my own. And two, I tend to initiate a fair number of sexual activities with my current partner, the true love of my adult life. Following a checklist — whether dreamed up by *Cosmo* or your man — just never feels sexy. Making your own fantasies together, as a couple, does.

Having years of emotional distance from the whole ordeal with my ex also helped me realize what was getting to me about his sexual requests: they seemed to come from a preapproved list in *Maxim* magazine or something, the ultimate markers of commoditized female sexuality. I wasn't even sure he wanted them, per se, as much as he wanted to prove he could have them (the same way, I must admit, I'd wanted an engagement ring from him just to prove I'd won at life). This was borne out one day, late in our relationship, when I danced on the bar at Coyote Ugly (yeah, just like the movie) at his urging, and he seemed more embarrassed than exhilarated.

The fact that my more spontaneous expressions of sexuality, the ones that came from the real me and not some trussed-up hussy version of me, weren't enough for him degraded me doubly. If this sounds familiar to you — fake sexuality being forced upon someone while her genuine sexuality is devalued — that's because it's called *the society we live in*. I don't blame my ex, who was as young and dumb as I was, for ideas foisted upon each generation through everything from porn to ads to magazines.

But if you're wondering whether to shoot that amateur porn video or wear that chafing crotchless latex onesie or enter that stripping contest at the request of your loved one, make sure you — and he — really want it to begin with. And if not, maybe it's time to find a new lover whose fantasies you fulfill just by being you.

— *Jennifer Keishin Armstrong*

Questions to Ask Yourself About Feminism and the Bedroom

1. What do you like best about sex?
2. Where do sex and feminism overlap in your life?
3. What kind of partner do you currently want, if any? A casual-sex encounter, a fling, a friend-with-benefits, a mate for life? If you're not coupled, decide what you want and stick to it (unless and until what you want changes, of course). If you are coupled, make sure you're in the arrangement that best suits you right now.
4. What's one change that could make your current sex life better? Maybe it's just a better vibrator, or a new position with your partner, or a nightly erotic story.
5. When has sex made you feel the most guilty, and why?

Feminism in the Bedroom Action Plan

1. Examine your sexual history to determine what you like and don't like, on a fundamental level, regardless of what your partner at the time wanted or enjoyed. If you're single, look for a partner with tastes complementary to yours. If you're coupled, talk to your partner about your likes and dislikes so you're in sync moving forward.

2. Find your local female-centric sex-toy shop. Stock up on vibrators and lube and condoms and anything else you might enjoy; take a class; talk to the staff there. They're usually super-smart, very nice, and, most of all, the least judgmental people ever.

3. Complete a Yes-No-Maybe list, which you can find online. It's a checklist of sexual options you can complete either alone, so you're clear on your own desires and no-go zones, or with a partner. It's an easy, fun, liberating experience either way — trust us.

4. If you feel so inclined, investigate an alternative sexual lifestyle, like polyamory (check out Lovemore.com), BDSM (BDSMguide.org), swinging (Nasca.com), and others, just to see what's out there.

5. Write in your journal about your best and worst sex experiences of all time. You'll be surprised by what you remember, and what you learn.

6. Read Jaclyn Friedman's *What You Really Really Want* and do the exercises to find out what *you* really really want. There's no better way to improve your sex life and make it more feminist.

ELEVEN

FEMINIST RELATIONSHIPS: FROM LONG-TERM TO LIFELONG PARTNERSHIP

B ETTY FRIEDAN JUMP-STARTED feminism's all-important second wave when she lacerated housewifery with her move-ment-shaking book *The Feminine Mystique*. The book iden-tified "the problem that has no name" — essentially, overeducated women trapped in their homes with vacuums and ovens wonder-ing in bleak mass silence, *Is this all?* Friedan herself was married when she wrote it, to adman Carl Friedan (whom she later divorced and publicly accused of beating her). The idea for the book came in 1957, when Friedan took a survey of her fellow Smith graduates for their fifteenth reunion about how they'd used their college education: she found few of them had used it at all. Thus was born her groundbreaking look at middle-class women's mass ennui, and her indictment of wifehood as it stood.

More recently, Feministing.com founder and feminist author Jessica Valenti has spoken and written about her efforts to bring weddings and marriage into the modern age, sans sexism. It hasn't been easy. "As I soon learned, there is no such thing as perfect when you're a feminist getting married," she wrote, referring to the disappointment friends and family expressed with her lack of a romantic proposal story. She kept her last name, much to many family members' chagrin. "The fact that Andrew and I had had conversations about the misogynist traditions that accompany marriage made us a bit of an oddity, it seemed," she wrote. "Then there were the fellow feminists who felt that getting married was a sop to the patriarchy. . . . Because, with the best will in the world, kissing goodbye to gender roles can be more difficult than it looks." Therein lies the modern problem with no name. We'll call it something like debilitating feminist guilt over wanting to join your life with that of a wonderful, feminist guy while also wanting to maintain your own identity. It's not as catchy as the feminine mystique, but it's almost as vexing.

So what do we do? Vow never to fall in love with a man, much less get married? Let's face facts: heterosexual women are attracted to, and fall in love with, men. So we're stuck with them if we want love, sex, and babies. Sometimes during the course of all that, they might pay for dinner, and that's not a reflection on your feminism unless you're refusing to pull your weight in the relationship or he's refusing to allow you to participate in it.

Both genders win when feminism enters a relationship. Each party does nice things for the other out of love, caring, and compassion. Resentments don't fester for decades only to explode upon impact with one of the other spouse's midlife crisis. Everybody's name reflects who he or she is, and no one loses the person he or she was before the relationship began. No one feels taken advantage of or trapped. And the sex, as we discussed in our bedroom chapter, is great.

We need men to not only believe in our equality but also actively fight for it — what better way to get them on our side than to start at home?

It's almost too much to fantasize about, though: Is there such a thing as a feminist relationship that's also still romantic and sexy and fun? We say yes, *of course*, but you have to demand it from the start. That means no game-playing, no using sex as manipulation, no passive-aggressive wiles as advocated by many a relationship-advice book. (Please see our chapter on dating-without-rules for further suggestions.) Both you and he should be contributing equally to the relationship from the start — to your sex life, to your social life, and to your finances, from dinners out at the beginning to mortgages and investments later on.

You have to negotiate equality for yourselves as a couple; one of you might be better at socializing, while the other might make a lot of money, but both parties should be showing up for the relationship in one way or another. Of course, we're talking mostly about hetero relationships here — they're where feminism and patriarchy can nestle up in bed right there between you. Gay relationships should be equal too, of course; it's just that their equality or inequality doesn't take on the same political implications as straight relationships.

You're striving for a sense of balance, not a constant power play and not an excuse to cry "feminism" every time he wants to help you with your coat. If you're a solid couple, chivalry doesn't apply. You're just both nice to each other, which you should want to be anyway.

Differences between the sexes have been a running gag among humans for a great deal of recorded history. In the more recent centuries, science has been twisting itself into knots to back this up with evidence or to refute the entire idea with evidence. Either way seems to make a splashy little news item, right? (Little regard is given to the size, scope, or scientific rigor of these studies, particularly if they seem to prove something the media is eager to see proved.) So we have studies that chart our brain differences: Men have denser neurons in their temporal neocortex, the part of the brain that helps with emotional and social processes! Stop the presses! We have studies that prove our differences in sex drive: Yep, men want it more, and women are more complicated. (We are more sensitive to environment and context, it seems.) Men are also 7 percent taller than we are, in case you couldn't figure that out. And by the way, the oft-quoted statistic that men's brains are larger than women's? Well, they are, because men are larger, on average. If you compare the organ's weight to body mass, however, you get a different story — women's brains are slightly larger per pound of flesh, if you want to get into it.

The point here isn't to quote silly statistics that prove one or

Celebrity Women Whose Partnerships Allow Them to Shine

Gwen Stefani and Gavin Rossdale: Gwen's the lead singer of an otherwise all-male band, a solo artist, one of the best pop-rock songwriters of our time, and a fashion icon. Gavin was the big star when her band No Doubt opened for his band Bush in the '90s, but now he's Mr. Stefani to most of the world, and that's worked for their decade-plus of marriage.

Julia Roberts and Danny Moder: One of the most bankable actors in the world marries a good-looking, down-to-earth camera-man . . . didn't we see this in a Julia Roberts movie once? No matter, it's her real life now, and nobody seems to have suited her better.

Oprah Winfrey and Stedman Graham: The Queen of Media — she'll always be that to us, talk show or no — has built her monstrous career over the past quarter century with the quiet support of her partner, Graham, an entrepreneur who stays behind the scenes. The pair got engaged in 1992 but decided to eschew marriage and its trappings for longtime commitment. And as far as we can tell, Graham has been the quintessential good man behind a great woman.

the other gender is superior; it's to say people are all different, and if you group them up and measure stuff, you can draw some sweeping conclusions, but they don't mean much in the context of one-on-one relationships. You need to throw all talk of gender differences out the minute you fall for someone (or preferably before) and focus on the specific man you've fallen for.

If you have used your *feminist*, not your feminine, wiles to land a good guy — and of *course* you have, or why would you be committing to a relationship with him? — you must declare, once and for all, that men are not the enemy. Relationships leave no room for battles of the sexes, at least not the kind of respectful, enriching relationships most of us say we want these days. Women must realize men do not inherently suck, contrary to many a drunken gab session with girlfriends. Do some men suck? Of course! (See Charlie Sheen, Anthony Weiner, Arnold Schwarzenegger, etc.) So do some women. But we must stop blaming everything that goes wrong in relationships on the alleged shortcomings of an entire gender. We have to be on their side when they deserve it, just as we want them to be on our side.

Sexy Feminist: Michelle Obama

The old expression "Behind every great man stands a great woman" is a lesson in condescending sexism. But in the case of First Lady Michelle Obama, it finds a new, feminist meaning.

Before she even met Barack, Michelle was an icon in the making. When she was growing up on the South Side of Chicago, her family was short on cash but rich on ambition. Michelle's father set high standards for his kids, both of whom attended Princeton as undergrads. Michelle then went on to receive her JD from Harvard, where she made a name for herself on campus for organizing demonstrations calling for more minority students and professors.

She returned home to Chicago, and she rose through the ranks of the law firm where she met Barack (she was *his* mentor), then worked for Mayor Richard M. Daley and the University of Chicago Medical Center. Meanwhile, she married Barack and had two daughters. She epitomized the "have it all" woman: high-powered career, an equal marriage, and motherhood. She also prioritized her personal values. She left her lucrative career in corporate America to go into public service, advocating on behalf of women, children, and young adults. She put into action the lessons she taught her children — that public service makes you a better person, diversity makes this a better society, and everyone deserves a chance to live a healthy life.

Every move she makes is fueled by personal passion. She doesn't have to shout that she's a feminist to show us she is one. When the president speaks of Michelle, he talks of her strength, drive, and dedication to the welfare of all. This isn't just rhetoric but a life's mission she's invested in — and one that helps influence policy that affects all of our lives. There's nothing more feminist than that.

Not since Jackie Kennedy has there been so much attention paid to a First Lady's fashion sense. But Michelle Obama brings a fresh element of "real" to her image: she's been photographed wearing couture gowns and J. Crew twin sets and feels at home in both.

She also has the figure of a healthy woman rather than a rail-thin fashion plate. The media's coverage of her style reflects the importance of this. Rather than focusing on her sexuality, discussions about Michelle Obama's look concentrate on her strength:

Those arms! Those calves! She's comfortable in her own skin, she owns her athletic build, and she encourages other women to do the same. It's no wonder so many American women have made her their fashion icon. She sets an achievable standard.

Loving and supporting your man is a feminist act. Michelle Obama demonstrates just that. It's clear that Michelle and Barack Obama adore each other. Michelle doesn't shy away from valuing and admiring her husband, a positive message to all women. The sooner we realize men can be our greatest allies in the fight for equality, the sooner that fight ends. The First Lady doesn't shy away from letting her opinions be heard either. The 2011 biography *The Obamas* reveals how influential Michelle has been in hiring and firing close aides and strategists, keeping the president focused on his key legislative goals, and holding him (and the entire executive staff) accountable for values.

Marriage may be rooted in patriarchal women-as-chattel customs, but that's no longer what it has to stand for today. It's about partnership and family, two values essential to fighting any inequality. Michelle's clear devotion to her husband and his vision for the country is to be admired, not criticized. Granted, she's also reportedly chafed at the constraints of White House life and the demands of being a ladylike First Lady, but she's faced the challenges of balancing feminist self-determination and support of her spouse with remarkable public grace. In the process, she's shown women that choosing to prioritize your family's goals, which sometimes may mean focusing on the husband, over your personal ones is courageous. We dream of having the chance to vote for her someday.

Presuming you've landed this wonderful man — an enlightened man who isn't aggressive or abusive or controlling — negotiating a long-term committed relationship to him without encountering feminist roadblocks can still be challenging. He may not turn out to be a perfect-angel-male-feminist 100 percent of the time. And being with him may require compromises that make you *feel* a *tad* bit unfeminist, but then again, does it have to do with feminism or just with being in a normal relationship? Normal relationships require compromise no matter what, right? So there you are, stunned into complete inaction over something like whether you should wash the dishes even though it's his turn but he had a hard day, or fuming over what he meant when he said you'd look good in the too-short skirt you saw on a mannequin at the mall in the window of the teen-girl store.

And marriage exacerbates all this fretting, because marriage, of course, was traditionally viewed as a hierarchy — man on top, good wife supporting him. But feminism has done marriage some good, despite what many conservative activists will tell you: as women have made economic gains, the divorce rate has fallen. Several studies have shown a link between shared housework and more sex for married couples.

These statistics suggest it *is* possible to redefine traditional gender roles. Plenty of partnerships now survive the woman outranking the man career wise, according to a Pew survey. "There are relationships that are complementary, in which each person feels like they have their own sphere," says Michael Kimmel, coauthor of *The Guy's Guide to Feminism*. "Then there are relationships that are egalitarian, where they divide everything equally. Then there are feminist relationships. They don't just split everything, but they talk about it. It's not enough to just make it a personal decision to share everything; you have to see those decisions as political. . . . It requires effort."

For many of us, having equal relationships means *we* have to be the ones to adjust — to the idea of doing our share of traditionally female tasks like housework and child care, ideas we've spent our lives railing against. "I clean the house," feminist singer-songwriter Ani DiFranco told writer Jennifer Baumgardner in a 2011 interview. "My mother was an early feminist. She was outraged to be doing all the housework, taking care of the children, and cooking when she got home from work. I inherited her outrage, and that righteous anger has been a part of my art and my growth. Coming back around to standing at the sink, doing dishes *without* outrage, has been a long journey for me."

Feminist Confessions: Compromise in Marriage Doesn't Mean Throwing Out Feminism

I have some confessions: I make dinner for my husband, I added his name to mine (no hyphen), and I am the primary caregiver for our son. And, yes, I am a feminist in a feminist-leaning marriage. What does that mean? It means real life sometimes doesn't allow for a perfect combination of empowerment and responsibility. It's a relationship that requires compromise — sometimes more difficult than you'd ever imagined — to make things work. As is the case for so many heterosexual couples, my husband makes more money than I do, works in an industry that demands more of his time outside of the home, and carries fewer of the domestic responsibilities. But we make it work, feminism intact. Here's what I learned from some of my own compromises:

Feminists make dinner too — even if we don't like to. I am a domestic goddess of the most reluctant variety. When I lived alone, I used my refrigerator to store beauty products and never once turned on my oven. Now that I'm married and a mom, grabbing sushi and smoothies are not practical options. There are three of us who need to eat, and I have chosen to take on the responsibility of making sure we eat well.

My husband would never expect me to be a "dinner's ready, honey" kind of woman, even if I liked to cook. He's evolved like that. But he definitely prefers homemade food over taking a trip to Wienerschnitzel because I couldn't get dinner together. That brings up another point: Wienerschnitzel? Yeah, my dear man's go-to self-fending food is often of the fast, greasy, and surely life-shortening kind. When he eats what I prepare, he gets leafy greens, organic meat, and whole grains. While I don't know if I'll ever love cooking, I will always be a food snob. I prefer — mandate, actually — healthy, unprocessed food. So I balance the burden of cooking with the joy I get from my weekly trips to the farmers' market, watching my son devour organic avocados and knowing that I am helping my family lead a healthier life. But we order takeout at least once a week.

Cleaning sucks. No one likes washing dishes, scrubbing toilets, or emptying lint traps. My husband and I divide these chores between us the best we can, but because he works about twelve

hours a day and I work from home (whether writing or baby-wran-
gling), the bulk of these tasks falls on my shoulders. This is crazy-
making. Before we had a child, I used to spend entire Saturdays
(when he worked weekends) cleaning the house and resenting the
hell out of him when he got home because I'd spent my day off
doing chores rather than with my friends or doing things for myself (I feel Ani DiFranco's rage at the kitchen sink). Now that we
have a kid, I have no days off, and the cleaning is constant. Solution: housekeeper! This is no longer an indulgence for the rich
and famous. Friendly, reliable cleaning professionals are affordable and may be the investment that saves your marriage. During
times when we couldn't find or afford one, I asked any babysitters
to also do some light cleaning and learned to live with a little bit
more mess than I'd prefer. I'll ignore that sink full of dirty dishes
if it means I can have twenty minutes to myself with a book and
some tea.

Money talks: Ugh. Some of us have our debt demons, and
they come shrieking out of the closet when you get married. This is
never easy, but one of the hardest lessons my husband and I both
learned is that we have to come clean as soon as possible. We
know what we have to work on together and have established a
common savings goal. We have both joint and individual bank accounts and, by virtue of family budgeting sessions, hold each other
accountable for expenditures that are a bit too frivolous or irresponsible. Neither of us likes to be told what to do, but this system
of checks and balances is key to maintaining transparency (essential) in our marriage.

I have a new name, but I'm still the same person. He didn't want me to change my name; I ultimately did. I understand the oppressive history of this custom, but I weighed it against the other priorities in my life and marriage. His name was given to him by an adoptive parent so he was never that attached to it; it wasn't a bloodline to him, just a name. But from the time I met him, he expressed his desire to have his own biological family to feel the genetic connection he lacked growing up. I wanted to not only procreate with him but share an identity that means something as a family.

— *Heather Wood Rudúlph*

And yet, even in the most feminist relationships, reminders of patriarchy lurk in every corner. Let's begin with the wedding. On the one hand, tradition can be nice, making one feel like part of human history and part of one's own culture. That's what ceremonies are for, after all. And yet modern American cultural traditions for weddings are nothing short of a feminist minefield. First, there's the dress: white, of course, to signify your virginity! A veil, of course, to really get the virgin message across. Daddy giving you away to your husband. In some traditional Christian ceremonies, vows to obey. "I now pronounce you man and wife. You may kiss the bride." Even when you get to kiss, the man gets all the agency! All this, even as magazines tell you over and over that this is "your" big day.

The wedding is just the beginning of a long list of life adjustments that come with matrimony. Joint bank accounts, for starters. If you make more than he does, a man — even an otherwise enlightened one — will struggle with feelings of inadequacy and, worse, will know he's wrong and so won't talk about them. If you make less than he does, though, you're probably in for five times more angst (our unscientific estimate) than he'd ever experience in the same situation, thanks to the ever-present feminist guilt. He'll generously tell you he's happy to share his wealth with you, that all that cash in the account belongs to both of you now. But you will likely feel overpowered, unable to, say, do something as simple as buy new lip gloss if you want it because *why should he pay for your lip gloss?* But how *are* you supposed to buy lip gloss now? Do you have to ask him for permission? That doesn't seem right. But what is?

All this lip gloss business, of course, sidesteps the larger issue at stake: What if he decided to leave you? Or what if you wanted to leave him? Would you be left with nothing? Would you have the resources to leave him if, God forbid, things went awry, with your meager finances swallowed up in your shared account and no assets to show for it? It can make you feel like a kept woman, or it can make you feel trapped. In any case, it can make the marriage feel inherently unequal, a bad place to be.

"I don't think there's a perfect type of marriage," says Pamela Haag, who charts the history of modern matrimony in her book *Marriage Confidential.* "However, there is a perfect *state* of marriage, and that state is fairness. To me, the ideal marriage is one in which the 'dreariness quotient' is in balance: Both partners feel as if they're each doing enough of the unglamorous, life maintenance work to keep the household and marriage humming, so that the marriage feels fair. In some ways, fairness is the final frontier for a feminist marriage."

Then there's the doozy of them all, the proof — in case we needed any — that marriage was designed as men's domain. Should you take his name? Though the history of the name-change tradition is hard to pin down, it seems to go back about as far as the use of surnames does, around a thousand years or so. When the use of last names came into everyday use, women's changing them upon matrimony signaled perhaps the most important thing in those days: the transfer of property from one family to another. Because women were bargaining chips that came with dowries, for the most part, they took their husbands' names. (Exceptions were occasionally made when the woman's family was significantly more powerful than the man's, thus making her last name more advantageous in old aristocracies.)

About 90 percent of brides in the United States still change their names to their husbands' upon marriage, each woman essentially changing her identity to join her life with her spouse's. Practical reasons to do this abound: so it's clear from your names that you're husband and wife, so your last name matches that of your children, and so joint checking account paperwork goes more smoothly. It also makes you and your new husband a family unit. Since this is kind of the point of getting married, it makes sense. More practical-minded women, even radical-feminist-minded ones, have seen the name-change tradition as a chance to escape their own long-despised given surnames. A friend of ours and writer for our site, SexyFeminist.com, who often serves as our hard-core-feminist reality check, couldn't fill out her name-change documents fast enough when she got hitched a few years ago: gone was her old byline, Alessandra Djurklou; she could now rebrand as the sleeker, easier-to-spell A. K. Whitney. "I really agonized over the name change, particularly since Djurklou is a very old and aristocratic name," Whitney says. "I was, technically, the Baroness Alessandra Katarina Djurklou. The fact that I married a commoner is still a teensy disappointment for my mom, ironically herself a commoner. But it occurred to me that I was just trading one man's name for another, and this new man was the kind, good, ethical man I truly admired. So the choice became easier."

However, nothing brands you with ownership more than subsuming your lifelong identifier — your own family's name, the name under which you may have built a career and a reputation — to your husband's. You could see keeping your name as a political statement, a stance against an old-timey tradition on par with the part of the wedding vows about obeying your husband. Or you could just see it as a practicality: Who wants to go through the trouble of changing your work e-mail address and your business cards and informing all kinds of people whose business it is not that you have decided to make a lifelong commitment to a man?

Suffragist Lucy Stone brought national attention to the issue in the mid-1800s when she became the first woman in American recorded history to retain her maiden name after marrying (she married abolitionist and Republican Party cofounder Harry Blackwell). The Lucy Stone League, a group that continues to advocate for women to keep their names, puts it in stark terms: "When girls are growing up, they see what they have to look forward to: the abandonment of their identity into the identity of another. What incentive do they have to develop their full identities in their adolescence? In some prison cultures, inmates are given numbers and their names are taken from them. One purpose of this practice is to strip away a sense of importance and humanity from the inmates . . . the tradition of women giving up their names is equally damning."

Hyphenation gained prominence as the second wave took off in the 1970s, as did the movement for women to not be identified by their marital status with *Miss* and *Mrs.* designations. Hyphenation and combination names (think Hillary Rodham Clinton) remain well-known, but still shockingly uncommon, practices. Some couples have opted for both spouses to switch to hyphenated or combined names, with a few pioneers going so far as to elide their last names into a new one. A Taylor and a Jones we know became the Tayjos, for instance — the last-name version of tabloid couple nicknames like Brangelina.

Even after you've gotten through the basics of setting up your married life, you still face one key question: What does being a good wife mean when you're also a feminist? Few people still believe in the 1950s home-ec textbook model of having dinner ready for him when he returns from work, keeping a spotless home, soothing him after his hard day, and giving in to wifely bedroom duties. But that doesn't mean we should never participate in homemaking chores, nor does it mean we don't want to be good spouses — just as we hope our husbands will be. Recent studies have even shown that men crave romance — particularly cuddling — so you can't go wrong by giving your husband some good old-fashioned love. We can't think of *anything* unfeminist about that. The trick is making everything you do in the name of your marriage a conscious choice and always feeling equal to your husband.

Sexy Feminist Action Plan: Ten Ways Your Man Can Be a Feminist

1. By calling himself a proud feminist. We know there has been plenty of debate over whether men can even be considered feminists without the life experience of oppression to back it up — some argue they should be called pro-feminist — but we say no movement is going to get anywhere if it excludes half the population. When even lots of women deny their feminism, should we shut out men who embrace it?

2. By fighting for causes deemed women's issues, like sexual-assault awareness and education, reproductive rights, and domestic violence prevention

3. By supporting good female candidates for office as well as pro-woman candidates (these aren't always the same!)

4. By mentoring women in his field

5. By encouraging daughters' ambitions and sharing his passions with them — whether that's astronomy, chess, cooking, or decorating

6. By speaking up against men saying and doing sexist stuff

7. By giving you support and room to be the woman he fell in love with, no matter what

8. By commenting in online forums about his feminist stance. We need this to combat the overwhelming morass of disgusting attitudes online!

9. On that note, also by reading feminist sites, just to stay on top of the issues, if he's into that

10. By making sure he's giving you what you want, and not giving you what you don't want, in bed. Like we said, feminist sex is fun.

TWELVE

FEMALE FRIENDSHIP: THE ULTIMATE FEMINIST ACT

IN THIS BOOK, we've discussed dozens of ways media creations tear women down — impossible beauty standards, diet mania, slut-shaming, competition in the workplace. But these forces come with an undercurrent that wears away at the most important bonds in our lives: they divide us from other women, the very people who could help us fight such insidious ideas by talking about them and uniting against them. Beautiful women may garner certain benefits in our society, for instance, but they often lack many female friends because they inspire such insecurity in others. And nothing separates a group of women faster than an offer of dessert — some will want it, some will moan about their guilt, and others won't want it at all, but it's likely few of them will get through it without haranguing another for whatever her reaction to it is.

Stories about women's constant defects and failings is catnip to a media that has learned that women swallow these concepts whole and then rush to purchase products meant to fix them. Single and married women sniping in the press over whose life is better; the mommy wars that pit working mothers against the stay-at-homes; the "man shortages" that make us see one another as constant competition; the endless onslaught of judgment hurled online at famous women's bodies and clothes . . . it all adds up to dividing us to conquer.

But we *could* just as easily choose to conquer by uniting. Mary Wollstonecraft, who in 1792 wrote the proto-feminist manifesto *A Vindication of the Rights of Woman*, credited two female friends with her early intellectual development: Jane Arden, with whom she often read books and attended lectures by Arden's philosopher father, and Fanny Blood, with whom she envisioned an all-female utopia but more practically set up a school with her for Church of England dissenters. Wollstonecraft loved her female friends to possessive lengths. She once wrote to Arden: "I have formed romantic notions of friendship . . . I am a little singular in my thoughts of love and friendship; I must have the first place or none."

Janice Raymond's 1986 book *A Passion for Friends* shows how women throughout history have turned to female friends as partners in patriarchal resistance. From nineteenth-century marriage resisters in China, who refused matrimony by living together, to nuns who bonded over their spiritual ties and escaped from male-dominated life, women have had power in numbers. Raymond writes: "By blaring the hetero-relational message that 'women are each other's worst enemies,' men have ensured that many women will be each other's worst enemies. The obstacles to female friendship get good press. The message functions as a constant noise pollution in women's lives and is heard in many different places. Constant noise about women not loving women is supplemented by the historical *silence* about women always loving women."

For a modern case in point, take Jennifer Baumgardner and Amy Richards. The two met when they were co-underlings at *Ms.* magazine in the 1990s and turned their budding friendship into a joint book project, *Manifesta,* that would become a definitive work on third-wave feminism and would lead to another coauthored work, *Grassroots: A Field Guide for Feminist Activism.* "I've always been attracted to people who are what I call intellectual muses — i.e., people who provoke creativity and productivity in me," Baumgardner told us. "For Amy and me, who both had and have lots of ideas and energy, we clicked over affirming the other person's ideas and getting excited about them. The first big project was writing *Manifesta* — a book we wrote in our twenties. We had to learn how to write a book together, and we each brought different strengths that usually complemented one another. Writing a book is really difficult and tedious, but also tremendously gratifying — so we had each other to share both the hard times and the glory."

Adds Richards: "I think there is something to be noted about friendship and collaboration. I have many strong female friendships, and most of my friends have ended up in fields related to mine. We don't work directly together, but doing parallel works reaffirms both our friendship and our professional lives. And of course, what is at the root of a good friendship is what has to be at the root of a good working relationship — respect for who the other person is and what they uniquely bring to the table."

WOMEN GET FRIENDSHIP RIGHT THE FIRST TIME, THEN WE BREAK IT

Every girl falls in love for the first time with her best friend. This has nothing to do with sexual orientation and everything to do with the strength of female friendship. You meet cute in elementary school, maybe even sooner, and grow up together, sharing clothes, secrets, Popsicles, and boy crushes. You're inseparable. You beg your parents to let you sleep over at her house or let her sleep over at yours. She makes you light up when you're together, and when you get in a fight, it hurts in a way you're not sure how to describe; all you know is you want it to go away. You cry when she goes off to summer camp without you. You *sob* when you attend separate high schools. You write about her in your diary, as you will write years later about your first boyfriends.

Then somewhere around age fourteen everything changes. You're both getting boobs and attention from boys, most likely to different degrees. One of you gets a boyfriend, the other is busy with afterschool activities, and you don't see your first love as much as you used to. You either lose touch or stop talking, shooting awkward or mean glances at each other between classes because of hurt feelings or a fight you can't even remember. This is your first breakup — and broken heart.

Our first female friendships are so crucial to our emotional development that they can make us or crush us with one great sleepover talk or one party-invitation snub. We learn how to trust and love with these friends. We also learn the importance of honesty, loyalty, and forgiveness. So why is it that deep, binding love so quickly turns into competitive angst when we hit puberty? Kelly Valen spent twenty years as a lawyer and became a mother of four before she realized she'd been running from female friendships most of her life. A date rape in college followed by a slut-branding and ousting by her sorority sealed her fate; she never felt close to women again. Part epiphany, part therapy, her book *The Twisted Sisterhood: Unraveling the Dark Legacy of Female Friendships* examines the ways in which women destroy one another, often in the name of sisterhood. "We women swim in shark-infested waters of our own design," she wrote in the *New York Times* in 2007. "Often we don't have a clue where we stand with one another — socially, as mothers, as colleagues — because we're at once allies and foes."

If we bond and love one another based on emotional and psychological need, then we must fight when things get in the way of that essential relationship. What drives many women apart is competition — for a man, a job, or one another's attention. Men: we love them! And we're supposed to — they are the other half of the human race, necessary for our survival and biologically designed to be our mates (for those of us biologically designed to desire men). But somewhere along the line, someone decided men were more important than women, and we've been fighting that unequal standard ever since.

Rather than uniting women, this imbalance seems to drive women farther apart. Women at work feel pressure to compete.

When a certain kind of woman attains a position of power, rather than lifting up her sisters, she steps on them to get ahead, not knowing she's only hurting herself. Mothers share an emotional and experiential bond that should make their friendships rock solid, yet the judgmental, negative mommy chatter that thrives on-line, in playgrounds, and behind backs is worse than the sniping of a pack of mean girls in high school.

And when it comes to dating and love, women can be most brutal. Yes, it's a cliché to point fingers at men for driving women apart, and yet, it happens. But let's look at *why* it happens. Rarely is it the movie version — man falls for the mean girl; his sweet, supposedly mousy friend (she looks something like Julia Roberts) pines for him; and when the mean girl is revealed for who she is — ta-da! — true love prevails! This common story arc is both fantastical and derogatory. It tells us: Ladies, your Prince Charming is out there — maybe right under your nose! — you just have to beat the bitch to the punch to snag him. This message of snagging a man (as if there were nothing more important to do on the planet) is pounded into our little developing emotional heads from childhood (Barbie + Ken = Dream Life!), to adolescence (*Twilight* and almost every teen-targeted book, film, and TV show ever created), and on to adulthood (the attention paid to celebrity and royal weddings and every how-to article in most major women's magazines). Almost all media promote the same message: What you wear, how you act, and — perhaps most important — how you seek to please a man determine your likelihood of finding one who will go ahead and marry you and thus give you all the happiness you've been longing for. These ideas are essentially telling us each this: as a single woman, you are not capable of being fulfilled, happy, or successful.

This desire — some might say instinct — to look for love and the yearning to be loved in return is neither wrong nor the thing that drives a wedge between women. It's the importance placed on romantic heterosexual relationships that does it. What would happen if the mousy Julia Roberts girl were instead kind to the mean girl and discovered a stronger relationship than that dude they were fighting over could ever have provided? A romance worth telling! But not the story popular culture supports — nor is it the narrative we're taught from an early age.

In fact, there's such a societal pressure for women to be partnered with men that if two ladies form a bonded, meaningful relationship — not unlike the BFFs of our childhood — they're assumed to be either secretly gay, man-haters, or social pariahs (because clearly a woman isn't normal if she's not dating, married, or at least regularly fucking a guy). One of our feminist Twitter friends, Allison, is an example that illustrates both sides. Allison is a smart, articulate, hilarious woman in her late twenties who happens to cite her best friend as the most important person in her life. The two are the kind of buddies who are inseparable and often accompany each other as the designated "plus one," no matter the occasion. "She's done so many things for me just because, and I for her, and we know each other is there. That's just the way it is," she says.

Allison says some friends often mock them, cast glances that imply *Oh, the poor girls don't have dates*, or not-so-jokingly suggest they go ahead and partner up as lesbian lovers. Their closeness even caused a rift between the two of them and their third roommate — something Allison describes as "jealous weirdness." "I believe it's because neither of us are involved with a gentleman type," she says. "I've gone on a couple of dates, and so has she, but neither of us have had a significant relationship since we've been room-mates. Personally, I'm okay with that — more now than when I was younger — because I'm not the type of person who will go seek-ing out a man just to say I have one. If something happens with the different things going on in my life, great, but I keep busy on my own. But the idea that because I do happen to spend time with and have kinship with another lady means that we're a romantic couple is just offensive to me. My friendship with her is greatly im-portant to me — why should I stop spending time with someone who means a lot to me and whose company I enjoy because it's not the kind of relationship that is supposed to be our 'end goal'?"

Why, indeed? With the pressure to partner with men so per-meating women's lives, a woman can't win — she's either compet-ing for a guy or not doing her job as a normal gal if she shares unabashed closeness with a female friend. Some sociologists ar-gue that women have been socialized to express aggressive actions through indirect means — using behavior such as shunning, stig-matizing, and gossiping to emotionally cripple those standing in the way of the achievement they seek. (See chapter 7 for more on that.) Love and friendship are both part of the competitive sport fe-male relationships have become.

THE TRUTH ABOUT FEMALE FRIENDSHIP: REALITY IS BETTER THAN FICTION

If we look at representations of female friendships in popular cul-ture, the picture is bleak. The go-to model seems to be catfight as central plot line: *Real Housewives*, whether in New York, New Jersey, or Atlanta — or wherever else they're popping up now — make sport out of women tearing one another down. They compete and compare the wealth and worth of themselves and their husbands. They try to one-up one another for the Most Dramatic Episode Ever (more points if things are thrown or broken), and they play at being friends one day, then whisper and snicker behind one another's backs the next. Yes, this is manufactured reality TV, but why is this the model for rich, famous, and fabulous the country became hooked on? There have been half a dozen iterations of this show with no signs of them stopping.

Romantic comedies don't often do us favors either. *Bride Wars*, in which two best friends both get engaged: Eek! OMG, so happy for each other! But oh no! — they have the same wedding date and want the same wedding venue, and all of a sudden it's a one-up-manship feud that escalates to hair-pulling and frosting-throwing. Sigh . . . Even less extreme offerings, such as *My Best Friend's Wedding*, pit women against each other.

Positive Examples of Female Friendships in Pop Culture

Not all depictions of female friendships in entertainment are skewed. These examples showcase the best, the worst, and — best of all — the truth about female friendships.

Bridesmaids: This film not only gave the manicured middle finger to the no-girls-allowed comedy club but also showed female friendship in its real, raw, honest state. We fight, we make up, we occasionally resent each other, but at the end of the day we each know we're not complete without the other.

Mary Tyler Moore: Mary Richards is a beloved feminist icon for showing us a career woman who dared to be single — and love it. But perhaps the strongest thing about this show is the friendship between Mary and Rhoda. The two opposites — Mary's a quintessential midwestern good girl, Rhoda's a brash gal from the Bronx — start out fighting over the same apartment in the first episode, but by the second they're scouting the singles scene together, and their bond is rarely threatened from then on.

The Golden Girls: Four women who have had their marriages, families, and careers spend their twilight years together, happier than ever. The combination of Rose's sweet innocence, Blanche's unabashed sexuality, Sophia's hilarious snark, and Dorothy's stable, unifying reason is a perfect marriage — no men required.

Oprah and Gayle: Even the most influential woman on the planet needs a confidante. It's no wonder the one relationship Oprah shares with the public is the one she has with her best friend, Gayle King. In segments on Oprah's show, in interviews, and in public appearances, the two light up whatever space they inhabit. They joke, quarrel, cry, and support each other like sisters, and their strength and solidarity is something we could all learn from.

Sex and the City: With all its glitter and fantasy, *SATC* was real in its depiction of die-hard female friendships. These four women — so different it's astounding they're BFFs in the first place — fought, feuded, loved, lost, and stayed together through it all. *SATC* was strongest when it showed this foursome as a united front — rallying in support when Miranda's mother died or Samantha had cancer, comforting Carrie after her Post-it breakup, and smacking down rude men making comments about Miranda's post-baby body. They also called one another on their shit, which is essential to honest friendship.

As longtime business partners who started out as friends, we know the bonding power of a common cause. Our shared purpose, exploring women's issues through our website, SexyFeminist.com, has kept us close through Heather's marriage and the birth of her baby, through Jennifer's calling off her wedding and juggling a demanding schedule of full-time jobs and book writing, and through seven years of living on opposite coasts. We continue to communicate almost every day via text, IM, e-mail, and phone. We talk as much about abortion rights and media portrayals of women as about man troubles and family drama.

We stumbled upon this arrangement, and we consider ourselves damn lucky for it. Because we want to share that luck, we urge women everywhere to find themselves their own version: Pick a cause — we have a handy list of many lady-oriented ones in the next chapter — and pick a friend with whom to tackle it. If we all support one another *and* champion women's greater good while we're at it, there's no telling how far we can go.

And *that* is Sexy Feminism.

Sexy Feminist Action Plan: Why Being a Good Friend Is Being a Good Feminist

1. **Understand that your expectations are not those of everyone else.** You went to an Ivy League school, but your best friend or sister has a trade license or works as an assistant. Don't assume she's miserable or unfulfilled. Everyone has the opportunity to forge her own path in life. Support your girls on theirs, no matter how different it is from your own.

2. **Be flexible.** Everyone's life has its own set of obligations. When you both were single, struggling assistants, you had a standing date for martinis and movies on Mondays. Now that one of you has children or a fancy new job, adjust your expectations.

3. **Be dependable.** Just because your life is different from your friend's does not make it more important. Respect her by valuing your time together, showing up on time when you're scheduled to meet up, and calling her back.

4. **Understand that friendship changes, but you don't have to.** There are major changes in life that can cause friends to drift apart — when one gets married, has a child, gets a major promotion, or moves away. Each of these occasions is cause for celebration for your friend, no matter how hard it is on you to cope with how different your lives have just become. To make the friendship work, talk to her as honestly as you always have. Ask her questions rather than making assumptions and understand that a new family or career may take

priority over your friendship for a while. That doesn't mean
it's lost or devalued, just different.

5. **Make efforts to understand her life.** Get to know her husband, offer to babysit her kids, ask informed questions about
   her new career. Though you may not share as much in common as you once did, you can still be a great source of emotional support.

6. **It's not all about you.** A good friend will listen to the minutiae
   of your life over and over again and give as much attention
   to analyzing you as she does herself. But don't get greedy.
   If you have an especially attentive friend, remember that she
   needs to unload on you sometimes too.

7. **Know when to say when.** Not all friendships are made to
   last. If you've had consistently negative experiences with another woman, get sweaty palms at the thought of interacting
   with her, and feel empty after every new get-together, perhaps it's time to pull the plug on this friendship. Part of the
   beauty of being an adult is the free will to choose your own
   friends. Keep those who enrich your life and reciprocate your
   friendship efforts and lose those who drain you.

8. **Love your mother.** She's your first best friend, like it or not.
   This is the woman who made you into the person you are today. The next time you're urged to snap at her or roll your
   eyes, thank her instead.

ACTIVISM IS SEXY: REAL WAYS TO FIGHT FOR FEMINISM

T HROUGHOUT THIS BOOK we've suggested ways for you to apply the principles of feminism to your daily life without breaking too much of a sweat. Now it's time to break that sweat. Being an activist feminist can be just as easy as buying one lipstick brand over another; the work is in the thoughtfulness of every decision you make. But it's important to understand that feminism extends beyond the choices women make for themselves; it's a social movement whose purpose is to fight for equality and fairness for all. Think of Gloria Steinem's update on the definition of feminism: not just believing in social, economic, and political equality for all, but doing something about it. The awareness we've been preaching throughout this book should extend to our sisters, brothers, neighbors, and the global community. Here are some ways to make feminist activism a part of your everyday life.

FIGHT FOR REPRODUCTIVE RIGHTS

Since its widespread use began, fifty years ago, birth control has been a feminist issue. It may well be the single feminist issue that holds the most sway over women's individual lives. It's the difference between a delicate career-family balance and a life of GEDs, low-wage jobs, and dead-end careers. It's the difference between unwanted single motherhood and a well-timed child supported by ample resources and a mature parent or parents. It can make or break loves, careers, and lives.

But it's easy to forget all of that when you're popping your pill and going about your business, or you're raising kids without worrying about how other women are taking charge of their fertility. If you value your right to that pill, though, or if you want to be able to stop having kids after a few, or if you want to make sure your daughter doesn't someday end up with an unwanted pregnancy (or your son doesn't end up with an unwanted child), it's a right for which you should be fighting, any way you can. If you're going to take up one major area of feminist activism, this is a good one — particularly in these politically divided times, when the right to birth control is under attack by politicians looking for a lightning-rod issue. The fraught year of 2011, and pre-election 2012, proved, thank goodness, that there are limits to how far anti-choice activists can push America: The "personhood movement" — which seeks to "protect the pre-born" by establishing conception as the moment a person exists and thus brand everything from IUD use to abortion as murder — failed to pass a proposed constitutional amendment in Mississippi. Throughout 2011, conservatives rallied to defund Planned Parenthood, and longtime supporter the Susan G. Komen Foundation withdrew its grants to the organization. But public outrage won out. After a massive backlash, Komen reversed its decision. And following a nearly four-year battle, the Supreme Court made the Affordable Care Act law in June 2012. It provides the most progressive women's health coverage to date, granting women access to mammograms, cancer screenings, prenatal services, and free birth control. But just months prior, the Obama administration had overruled an FDA decision that would have allowed teenagers access to Plan B emergency contraception.

Being an activist for this issue takes paying attention and demanding more from your government and communities. Stay up to date on local and national legislation and understand what your vote means. Don't find yourself someday being denied your pills by a pharmacist who wants to make your life decisions for you, or paying exorbitant prices for it because your insurance doesn't cover it, or telling your daughter you can't afford protection for her because you were too busy to notice.

Don't be fooled by morality arguments either — you know, that contraception is akin to abortion, that it separates sex from reproduction, and that it encourages extramarital sex. Even 80 percent of anti-choice Americans think women should have access to birth control, according to a National Family Planning and Reproductive Health Association poll. If those pharmacists asking for a "conscience clause" truly wanted to keep people from preventing conception, they'd refuse to sell condoms too. If our society wanted men to take responsibility for contraception, it would have a male birth control pill. Restricting birth control is about controlling women's sexuality, about making women the perpetual sexual gatekeepers. It is, in short, about ingrained sexism.

That's what makes it both an age-old feminist fight and one worth caring about. While the endless abortion debate gets all the attention, family-planning services suffer in the crossfire. It's a cause every woman, regardless of politics — and even, perhaps, regardless of her stand on abortion itself — should get behind.

Action Plan

- Support NARAL and Planned Parenthood and similar organizations fighting to ensure that all women have access to safe reproductive medical care. Donate, volunteer, patronize, or blog to keep the rally alive.

- Stay up on reproductive rights debates in politics, and contact your representatives to support better sex education, access, and funding for all. And when you go to the voting booth, bring with you the knowledge of where candidates stand on reproductive rights. Support those who support your right to choose.

- Take control of your own reproductive rights by choosing methods that are right for you and talking to your partner or partners about your decisions.

- Support thorough sex education in schools that goes beyond abstinence. We owe it to our youth to give them the truth about sexual responsibility and to help them protect themselves.

BE A ROLE MODEL FOR YOUNG GIRLS

If feminism is going to thrive and survive, we need to offer the next generation better role models than Kim Kardashian and Snooki. There's no shortage of women whom teens can look up to, but these teens need help seeing them. Being an example yourself is a great start. If you have a chance to interact with girls (and if you don't, volunteer!), be an example for them. Talk to them about math, science, politics, and the world, not Ke$ha's new video (though starting off with that to break the ice is fine too). They may look up to you because of the cool shoes you wear, but use that as an opportunity to discuss how you worked hard to earn the money to pay for them. Foster their talents, feed their curiosity, and ask them about their dreams — girls need reminders every day that their dreams can come true.

And they can. Research shows that mentored teens are 46 percent less likely to start using drugs; 59 percent of kids improve their academic performance when mentored; and 73 percent become more goal oriented. Mentoring reduces the number of high-school dropouts, increases teens' likelihood of going to college, and improves their sense of discipline and self-esteem. Giving as much of your time and support as you can to young girls will help keep these statistics going in the right direction. There are countless organizations and nonprofits that need volunteers and mentors — you can visit mentor.org for opportunities near you. Here are a few of our favorites:

GEMS: Girls Educational & Mentoring Services serves girls and young women who have experienced commercial sexual exploitation and domestic trafficking. Through counseling, social programs, and mentoring programs, GEMS helps these young women and girls exit the sex trade and build new lives and confidence. **Gems-girls.org**

Professional Leaders of Women and Girls: Utilizes volunteers in professional sectors ranging from business to education in order to influence, inspire, and empower young girls of color. **Plwg.org**

Write Girl: Fosters creativity and self-esteem through intensive writing workshops aimed at showing teens that their voices matter. **Writegirl.org**

Big Brothers Big Sisters: With a chapter in nearly every city, BBBS has been proving the positive power of role models since 1966. **BBBSOS.org**

Girl Talk: Teaches leadership skills to teens by placing them in one-on-one mentoring relationships with their peers. Giving girls the tools to create their own positive self-images is a cause worth supporting. Chapters around the country need advisers, volunteers, and donors. **Desiretoinspire.org**

TAKE CARE OF THE EARTH

Why is environmental activism a feminist cause? At its core, feminism is about humanitarianism. Everyone must do her part to ensure a brighter future for the global population. Consider a few recent examples of natural disasters:

The 7-magnitude earthquake that hit Haiti in 2010 was the nation's most devastating in two centuries, not for its force but for the insurmountable destruction. This already-struggling country was not equipped to take the brunt of such a tremor, which resulted in the cities crumbling. The death toll of 300,000 and more than 2 million left homeless was the first blow. The unthinkable crimes against women (rape, beatings) and children (abandonment, illegal trafficking) that followed was the violent aftermath.

Bangladesh has one of the highest rates of starvation in the world — more than 40 percent of its residents are classified as malnourished, and 45 percent of all children are starving. This nation is one of the poorest on the planet, and it also has a history of natural disasters — tropical floods, cyclones, tornadoes, and monsoons hit every year. In 2007, Cyclone Sidr killed nearly 10,000 people and caused a whopping $1.5 billion in damage — about 2 percent of the nation's gross domestic product.

Even when disaster strikes industrialized nations — such as the 2010 earthquake and tsunami in Japan and the ongoing hurricanes and flooding in the southern United States — those that suffer most are families already living at or under the poverty line. Every time one of these environmental catastrophes strikes, humanitarian efforts are derailed, making already bad situations much worse.

In addition to donating to charities that fight against these atrocities, you have to live your life with respect to how it affects the environment. It matters.

Action Plan

Reduce, reuse, recycle. It's more than just a catchy slogan; it's something that should be a part of everyday life. Simple, consistent actions can make a world of difference — and just the difference the world needs to survive. Some ideas:

- We'd like to demand you never use another plastic bottle or grocery bag, but this is easier said than done. Invest in re-usable everything until you no longer need these items, and recycle anything and everything you can. Visit your county's website for details on everything that's recyclable. It's fascinating, surprising, and comforting to know how many things you can toss in the bin to be reused rather than piled in a landfill.
- Drive less.
- Walk more.
- Plant a tree or join a community garden.
- Clean out your closets twice a year and take your duds to a recycled-clothing store for credit, where you can buy new looks for way less. This is also a good way to shop when it's 90 degrees in December but retail stores are stocked with wool turtlenecks and fleece leggings. (This could be happening more, thanks to global warming.)
- Get crafty; create new uses for old things. We admit, we

suck at this, so enlist a crafty friend or children (they are *all* awesome at this) to help spark some ideas.

- Be a conscious consumer. If more of us buy consciously and demand better products from the corporations that sell us all the stuff we use, then that's what the marketplace will supply. That's how green cleaning products became mainstream and how the unfair, unsafe, and inhumane labor practices of some major manufacturers became public knowledge (visit Sweatfree.org for a directory of retail stores and companies that do not work with sweatshops). Every time you open your wallet, you're sending a message. It's an opportunity to speak up without saying a word.

Ten Feminist Charities That Need You

There are hundreds of charities for hundreds of worthy reasons; the world needs a *lot* of help. If you have a favorite to which you contribute, keep doing that. Here's a list of ten that are doing important feminist work. Visit the American Institute for Philanthropy (Charitywatch.org) for a more complete list of worthy charities, or research your own pet cause to find the best organization to help. You can even start your own.

Joyful Heart Foundation. Someone is sexually assaulted every two minutes in the U.S. One in three women reports being assaulted by a boyfriend or lover. Up to 10 million children witness domestic violence every year. These are staggering statistics. The fact that sexual assault and domestic abuse victims are often lost, sometimes forgotten, is even more enraging. This charity, founded by actress Mariska Hargitay, provides a safe haven for victims to heal, share, and move on with their lives. It also offers critical legal, mental health, and educational resources. **Joyfulheartfoundation.org**

UNICEF. The United Nations Children's Fund (formerly the United Nations International Children's Emergency Fund) was established to care for the millions of injured and displaced children in the aftermath of World War II. It has become the leading organization bringing food supplies to starving nations, educational opportunities to women and children, and lifesaving vaccinations and medical care to millions. Through all its efforts, it holds to the credo, "Aid is to be distributed without discrimination due to race, creed, nationality, status or political belief." **Unicef.org**

CARE. This charity's mission is simple: eradicate global poverty by empowering women and equipping them to survive and thrive. The focus is on giving women the tools to solve their own problems, thereby strengthening the communities in which they live and further empowering the next generations. The community-based charity works to improve education, prevent the spread of disease, increase access to clean water and sanitation, expand economic opportunity, and protect natural resources. CARE also delivers emergency aid to survivors of war and natural disasters and helps people rebuild their lives. Donate, volunteer, or find simple, social-media-based opportunities to support this important charity — like linking to it from your blog or Facebook page. **Care.org**

Global Fund for Women. This charity that works to eradicate poverty, discrimination, and crimes against humanity worldwide came about from a vision of three friends from Palo Alto, California. Anne Firth Murray, Frances Kissling, and Laura Lederer knew that women's human rights were central to making any real social, economic, or political change. They also knew that grassroots workers were the ones doing the most to make this change happen, but money is tight when you're a grassroots worker. Enter the Palo Alto three, who reach out to donors and pair their philanthropic contributions with the grassroots organizations changing the world. Since its inception, in 1987, the GFW has raised more than $85 million from donors, which has reached 4,200 groups in 171 countries. In 2010 alone, efforts reached 125,000 women and girls and benefited thousands more. These fabulous ladies prove that no idea is too small to make a reality — and everyone can make a difference. **Globalfundforwomen.org**

Save Girl Child. In India, thousands of little girls are born unwanted every year. In a society that values male heirs, hundreds of disappointed families name their girls Nakusa or Nakushi, both of which translate as "unwanted." Countless more are abandoned. A recent study revealed that couples in this country are having selective abortions to procreate only if the fetus is a boy, a practice some are calling gender-cide. This organization spreads awareness of this bias to the global community and seeks to empower women and encourage girls to believe in themselves and strive for greatness despite the obstacles they face. Funds raised help bring education to communities without it (UNICEF estimates that 65 million girls are out of school) and abolish forced child labor and child marriage. **Savegirlchild.org**

V-Day. This Eve Ensler–led charity is about more than just vagina love — a worthy cause in and of itself. Its mission is to end domestic violence against women and girls. Domestic violence is the leading cause of injury and death for women between the ages of fifteen and forty-four in the United States. Through benefits, performances of *The Vagina Monologues,* and campaigns led by women and college students, V-Day raises money for shelters (it opened the first ever in Egypt and Iraq), promotes domestic violence education, and has raised more than $85 million to protect and empower women worldwide. **VDay.org**

The White House Project. Hillary in 2008 was no fluke. There will be a female president in our lifetimes. But first, we need to encourage girls and young women to pursue careers in public service and politics — something they're often discouraged from doing. The WHP works to change that frame of mind by supplying women with the necessary tools to organize voting among women, adopt leadership roles in their communities, or run for office themselves. The website alone is such a treasure trove of nonpartisan resources and encouragement that it seems almost silly that we're not all making buttons that read VOTE FOR ME! **Thewhitehouseproject.org**

National Partnership. Fighting for better health care, support for working mothers (like never stopping until we get a national paid-family-leave policy), combating workplace discrimination, and speaking up when lawmakers vote against women's progress is a tussle we want to be in the middle of. So should you. **Nationalpartnership.org**

RAINN. A familiar voice on college campuses (we fondly remember participating in rape-awareness rallies sponsored by RAINN), this organization is as important now as it was when Tori Amos cofounded it, in 1994. The Rape, Abuse and Incest National Network is now the nation's largest anti-sexual-violence organization. Its hotline saves lives; its awareness campaigns save souls. And it doesn't work without volunteers. **Rainn.org**

Not for Sale. Slavery is alive and well across the globe, even in our own backyards. More than 30 million people in the world are subject to slavery — trafficked for sex, labor, . . . or worse. The most horrifying fact about this phenomenon is that it's hidden. NFS founder David Batstone was inspired to act when he read that female cooks at one of his favorite Indian restaurants in the California Bay Area were working as slaves, a story that came out after a deadly gas leak made the papers. His horror led to this charity that urges everyone to help end slavery first and foremost by talking about it (another icky thing we can't ignore). At the root of all of its volunteer efforts is education and information. Liking the organization on Facebook or tweeting about it may just be the spark that lights the fire for ten more people to get involved. We say that's a worthy twenty seconds of your time. **Notforsale.org**

GET LITERATE IN POLITICS AND MEDIA

No matter how well-read, politically educated, or media savvy you may be, the machines are still in the business of spinning. We could all use constant reeducation in understanding the inner workings of media and politics. Here's why:

Women and minorities are underrepresented in the media. We're a nation made up of 51 percent women and the majority race is no longer Caucasian, but the news media often focuses on stories that cater to a single demographic: white men. This is an issue that directly affects feminism. The media has the power to shape, influence, and change opinions. When women's and others' dissenting voices aren't a part of that conversation, they're left out of the change.

Marketing is manipulation. No matter how dignified and respectful the media organization, it has no choice but to sell you scripted, biased ideas and ideals right along with the news. Advertising dictates editorial copy in magazines (try to find an anti-wedding story in any American women's magazine — or even one in which the models aren't all wearing makeup). The big money in TV commercials influences news directors and programming executives to shape their programming to appeal to their sponsors (product placement, anyone?). News and entertainment websites give away your demographic information so that the right targeted ads pop up as you surf (how did they know you wanted a new pair of riding boots?). Understanding the ruse while consuming media is essential to not falling for it.

Action Plan

- Attend a media-literacy workshop or take a class at a local college. Use resources such as the Women's Media Center (Womensmediacenter.com) and the Center for Media Literacy (Medialit.org) to satisfy your curiosity and feed your knowledge base.

- For the love of freedom, vote! Millions of people are refused this right; it's irresponsible to squander it. Voting without knowledge, however, is worse than apathy.

- Distinguish between fact and mudslinging. Given the way that campaign ads use gossip, personal attacks, and hatred, you'd think they were written by the ultimate "mean girls." Don't believe everything you see — or read. Do your homework before voting.

- Talk about politics. Just as addressing issues of discrimination will force us to face the facts, debating the issues with anyone who can engage is the only way to a more open-minded society.

Political campaigns are games of rhetoric. It's easy to get caught up in campaigns, especially in an election year, which often feels like a long episode of *The Real World: DC* — complete with media-made archetypes and dramatic confessions. It's essential that we pay attention, but in the right way. Reading the newspaper, watching debates, attending town-hall speeches, and researching candidates all contribute to informed voting. But so, too, does understanding the bias in all of these. Knowing the issues at stake and where you stand on them will help you vote your convictions no matter who is running.

The amazing opportunities we have for activism are both inspiring and daunting. We know trying to pick the right one can be discouraging. The key to finding happiness — and continued success — in your activist work is to give your time to a cause that inspires and excites you. If you're a people person who loves talking to strangers, you may be perfect for collecting signatures for important civil rights campaigns. If you're a type-A organizer, a food bank or women's shelter may need your sorting skills. If you love to listen, work with the elderly. If you love to give advice, mentor young girls. The right fit for you is out there. The world needs you, and it deserves everything you have to give back.

APPENDIX

RESOURCES FOR SEXY FEMINISTS

SEXY FEMINIST READING LIST

Even though we don't agree with every one of these authors on every feminist issue, they all offer thought-provoking arguments particularly relevant to young women currently considering their own feminist beliefs:

Grassroots: A Field Guide for Feminist Activism by Jennifer Baumgardner and Amy Richards

Manifesta by Jennifer Baumgardner and Amy Richards

The Second Sex by Simone de Beauvoir

Full Exposure: Opening Up to Your Sexual Creativity and Erotic Expression by Susie Bright

APPENDIX: RESOURCES FOR SEXY FEMINISTS

The Hungry Self by Kim Chernin

Are Men Necessary? by Maureen Dowd

Pink Brain, Blue Brain by Lise Eliot

The Good Body by Eve Ensler

Backlash by Susan Faludi

Bossypants by Tina Fey

Losing It: America's Obsession with Weight and the Industry That Feeds on It by Laura Fraser

My Secret Garden by Nancy Friday

Women on Top by Nancy Friday

The Feminine Mystique by Betty Friedan

What You Really Really Want: The Smart Girl's Shame-Free Guide to Sex and Safety by Jaclyn Friedman

Marriage Confidential by Pamela Haag

The Guy's Guide to Feminism by Michael Kaufman and Michael Kimmel

Female Chauvinist Pigs by Ariel Levy

The Diet Survivor's Handbook by Judith Matz

I Can't Believe She Did That! by Nan Mooney

Fat Is a Feminist Issue by Susie Orbach

Women and Money by Suze Orman

A Passion for Friends by Janice Raymond

Unbearable Lightness by Portia de Rossi

Against Pornography by Diana Russell

The Twisted Sisterhood: Unraveling the Dark Legacy of Female Friendships by Kelly Valen

Full Frontal Feminism by Jessica Valenti

The Beauty Myth by Naomi Wolf

Vindication of the Rights of Woman by Mary Wollstonecraft

SEXY FEMINIST–MINDED WEBSITES AND BLOGS

Beautylish.com: An empowered take on beauty, makeup, and products

DodsonAndRoss.com: Betty Dodson, who was talking about women's orgasms and masturbation in the '70s when no one else was, and third-wave sex-positive feminist Carlin Ross offer a female-oriented, educational sex site. There's female-centric porn too.

Feministing.com: Political blog started by feminist author Jessica Valenti

Thefbomb.org: A feminist blog about women's rights for teen girls

TheFrisky.com: Women's lifestyle and entertainment site that goes beyond makeover and sex advice. It tackles weighty issues such as depression, feminism, and politics.

HotMoviesForHer.com: Pretty self-explanatory — porn for women!

Jezebel.com: *Gawker*'s female-oriented offshoot, with women's issues and attitude to spare

MyVag.net: Blogger Sarah writes with illuminating honesty about her, and all women's, lady parts.

Nerve.com: Intelligent, literary writing about sex

RookieMag.com: A fashion resource for teens and young women with a feminist bent, headlined by wunderkind Tavi Gevinson

SafeCosmetics.org: Tells us which beauty products are poisonous, which aren't

SexyFeminist.com: That's us!

VaginaVerite.com: "An unabashed exploration of the plain, ordinary, mysterious matter of vaginas"

REPRODUCTIVE RIGHTS

Center for Reproductive Rights (Reproductiverights.org)

NARAL (Naral.org)

Planned Parenthood Action Network (Plannedparenthoodaction.org)

MEDIA LITERACY

Center for Media Literacy (Medialit.org)

Geena Davis Institute on Gender in Media (Thegeenadavisinstitute.org)

Women's Media Center (Womensmediacenter.com)

WOMEN'S RIGHTS ORGANIZATIONS

Feminist Action Network (Feministactionnetwork.org)

Feminist Majority Foundation (Feminist.org)

National Organization for Women (Action.now.org)

NOTES

1. WHY FEMINISM IS SEXY

2   *Gloria Steinem's take on the word* feminist: Celina Hex, "Fierce, Funny, Feminists: Gloria Steinem and Kathleen Hanna," *Bust* 16 (Winter 2000): 52–56.

   "what our Paris Correspondent describes as a 'Feminist' group": Margaret Ferguson, "Feminism in Time," *Modern Language Quarterly* 65 (March 2004): 7–27.

3   *"mad, wicked folly"*: UK National Archives, http://www.nationalarchives .gov.uk/education/victorianbritain/divided/default.htm.

5   *"The enemy is not lipstick"*: Naomi Wolf, *The Beauty Myth: How Images of Beauty Are Used Against Women*, preface to revised paperback edition (1991; revised paperback edition New York: Anchor Books, 1992).

6   *"do-me" feminists*: Tad Friend, "Yes (Feminist Women Who Like Sex)," *Esquire* 121 (February 1994): 48–56.

   "bimbo" feminists: Maureen Dowd, "How to Snag 2,000 Men," *New York Times*, July 2, 1997.

   Immanuel Kant's categorical imperative: Immanuel Kant, *Grounding for the Metaphysics of Morals*, trans. James W. Ellington (Indianapolis: Hackett, 1993), 30.

10 *"Bitches get stuff done!"*: *Saturday Night Live*, NBC, first broadcast on February 23, 2008.

   "Bitch is the new black": Ibid.

   the New York Times *frets*: James C. McKinley Jr., "Vicious Assault Shakes Texas Town," *New York Times*, March 8, 2011.

11 *"a Liberated Woman"*: Gloria Steinem, "After Black Power, Women's Liberation," *New York*, April 4, 1969.

13 *"If you don't stand up for yourself"*: Marianne Schnall, "Interview with Gloria Steinem," Feminist.com, April 3, 1995, http://www.feminist.com/resources/artspeech/interviews/gloria.htm.

14 *"I stand on the shoulders"*: Sonia Sotomayor, "Full Text: Judge Sonia Sotomayor's Speech," *Time*, May 26, 2009.

2. OUR POOR VAGINAS

17 *"sexy vagina"*: Cover of *Cosmopolitan*, January 2010.
   millions who paused: "Blink and You'll Miss It," Lovefilm.com, February 24, 2011, http://corporate.blog.lovefilm.com/a-press-releases/blink-and-you%E2%80%99ll-miss-it.html.

18 *late '90s*: Ashley Fetters, "The New Full-Frontal: Has Pubic Hair in America Become Extinct?," *Atlantic*, December 13, 2011.
   crept into America in the 1950s: Denise Winterman, "Letting Your Hair Down," *BBC News Magazine*, January 12, 2007.
   hardest decision he'd ever made: Mark Steyn, "The Gubernator?," *Telegraph*, August 10, 2003.
   Brazilians hit U.S. shores: J. Sisters History, http://www.jsisters.com/site/.

19 *Gwyneth Paltrow, Kirstie Alley, and Jennifer Grey*: Christina Valhouli, "Faster, Pussycat, Wax! Wax!," Salon.com, September 3, 1999.
   Maxim vs. GQ circulation: Russ Smith and John Strausbaugh, "Maxim Dudes," *New York Press*, November 7, 2000.

20 Sex and the City *bikini-wax episode*: *Sex and the City*, HBO, September 17, 2000.

21 The View *bikini-wax episode*: *The View*, ABC, July 30, 2009.
   Grey's Anatomy *bikini-wax episode*: *Grey's Anatomy*, ABC, February 11, 2010.

23 *va-jay-jay*: *Grey's Anatomy*, ABC, February 12, 2006.
   Jennifer Love Hewitt unleashes vajazzling: *Lopez Tonight*, TBS, January 12, 2010.
   "Makes you sexy": Valhouli, "Faster, Pussycat."

24   *douching and pelvic inflammatory disease*: U.S. Department of Health
     and Human Services, http://www.womenshealth.gov/publications/
     our-publications/fact-sheet/pelvic-inflammatory-disease.cfm.

26   *two women hospitalized*: Beth DeFalco, "Brazilian Wax Ban?," AP,
     March 19, 2009.

27   *"Women are requesting the Brazilian"*: Salon worker, personal inter-
     view with Jennifer Keishin Armstrong, April 11, 2011.

29   *labial plastic surgery took off*: Shaun Dreisbach, "You Want a Prettier
     What?!," Glamour.com, April 1, 2008.

3. PLASTIC SURGERY: CAN YOU?

36   *sat down for a TV interview*: *Good Morning America*, ABC, May 11,
     2011; http://abcnews.go.com/Health/mom-year-daughter-botox-young
     -young/story?id=13580804#.UCssXGOe64Q.

37   *an IOU for breast implants*: "'Human Barbie' Sarah Burge Gives
     7-Year-Old Daughter Breast Implant Voucher," *Huffington Post*, June 9,
     2011; http://www.huffingtonpost.com/2011/06/09/human-barbie-boob
     -job-voucher_n_873705.html.
     breast implants and a nose job: Anderson, Warner Bros., November 29,
     2011.

39   *$10 billion industry*: "Report: Plastic Surgery a $10 Billion Dol-
     lar Industry in 2011," *PR Log*, March 21 2012, http://www.prlog
     .org/11830558-report-plastic-surgery-10-billion-dollar-industry-in-2011
     -with-92-million-procedures.html.

40   *"Let's face it"*: Haideh Hirmand, "What Happened to My Breasts? A
     Plastic Surgeon Explains," WOWOWOW, June 6, 2011, http://www
     .wowowow.com/lifestyle/what-happened-to-my-breasts-a-renowned
     -plastic-surgeon-explains/.

41   *220,000 plastic-surgery procedures*: "Teens and Plastic Surgery," Amer-
     ican Society for Aesthetic Plastic Surgery, October 12, 2011, http://
     www.surgery.org/media/news-releases/teens-and-plastic-surgery.

42   *incomes below $25,000 a year*: "2010 Plastic Surgery Statistics Re-
     port," American Society of Plastic Surgeons, http://www.http://www
     .plasticsurgery.org/Documents/news-resources/statistics/2010
     -statistics.

43   *Roughly 1 percent of women:* Average Breast Size Report, April 4, 2011,
     http://www.breastoptions.com.
     "definite certainty of implant failure": Website of Dr. Richard V.
     Dowden, last modified August 1, 2012, http://dr-dowden.com/main/
     augment.html.

45   *one of the highest mortality rates:* "Liposuction Deaths Higher Than
     Car Crash Fatalities," *Los Angeles Times,* November 13, 2007.

47   *80 percent since 2000:* Hallie Levine, "Would You Get a 'Mommy
     Tuck'?," *Redbook,* May 2011.

49   *2010 USC/Duke University medical study:* David T. Neal and Tanya L.
     Chartrand, "Embodied Emotion Perception: Amplifying and Damp-
     ening Facial Feedback Modulates Emotion Perception Accuracy," *So-
     cial Psychological and Personality Science,* published online April 21,
     2011.

4. VANITY IS NOT A FEMINIST SIN

55   *"checkmates women's attempts":* Naomi Wolf, new introduction to *The
     Beauty Myth: How Images of Beauty Are Used Against Women* (1991;
     repr. New York: Harper Perennial, 2002), 7.

57   *"the devil's making":* "Hair and Makeup," Erasofelegance.com, ac-
     cessed May 20, 2010, http://www.erasofelegance.com/fashion/makeup
     .html.

60   *"important power tool":* Beautylish.com biography of Erin Z., accessed
     March 2011, http://www.beautylish.com.

61   *"One of the things that defines us":* Vivian Diller, PhD, personal inter-
     view with the authors, March 2011.

63   *"There are no ugly women":* Helena Rubinstein, quoted in Nina Gar-
     cia, *The One Hundred: A Guide to the Pieces Every Stylish Woman
     Must Own* (New York: HarperCollins, 2008).
     2011 study proclaimed: Nancy L. Etcoff et al., "Cosmetics as a Fea-
     ture of the Extended Human Phenotype: Modulation of the Percep-
     tion of Biologically Important Facial Signals," *PLoS ONE* 6: e25656,
     doi:10.1371/journal.pone.0025656.

64   *$250 million worldwide:* MAC AIDS Fund, http://www.macaidsfund
     .org.

5. IS DIETING ANTIFEMINIST?

70 *eighty million Americans:* "America's Top 10 Healthiest Diets," *Health* magazine, last updated December 16, 2008, http://www.health.com/health/article/0,,20411397,00.html.

half of our population is considered overweight: "Adult Obesity Facts," Centers for Disease Control and Prevention, last updated August 3, 2010, http://www.cdc.gov/vitalsigns/AdultObesity/.

new epidemic: "Childhood Obesity Facts," Centers for Disease Control and Prevention, last updated June 7, 2012, http://www.cdc.gov/healthyyouth/obesity/facts.htm.

scary-ass truths: Harvard Eating Disorders Center, cited by Eating Disorder Foundation of Orange County, April 15, 2011, http://www.edfoc.org.

71 *"Ads for diets and dieting products":* Judith Matz, personal interview with the authors.

"Diets constrict women": Ibid.

73 *"emancipate themselves through slenderness":* "Fat Cats, Bodybuilders, and Corsets," by Sarah Stankorb, *American Magazine*, August 15, 2011, http://www.american.edu/americanmagazine/features/20110815-Vester-History-of-Dieting.cfm.

74 *more than $60 billion a year:* "U.S. Weight Loss Market Worth $60.9 Billion," PRWeb.com, May 9, 2011, http://www.prweb.com/releases/2011/5/prweb8393658.htm.

"the most potent political sedative": Naomi Wolf, *The Beauty Myth: How Images of Beauty Are Used Against Women* (1991; repr., New York: Harper Perennial, 2002), 187.

75 *"the media is such an incredible force":* Laura Fraser, personal interview with the authors.

76 *Carl's Jr. ads in the past decade:* Raphael Brion, "Slutburgers Gone Wild! Carl's Jr. Ads Through the Years," *Eater*, April 25, 2011, http://eater.com/archives/2011/04/25/slutburgers-gone-wild.php.

Gawker *coined the term* slutburger: Hamilton Nolan, "Padma Lakshmi in Sordid Bacon Cheeseburger Sex Tape," *Gawker*, March 26, 2009, http://gawker.com/5185737/padma-lakshmi-in-sordid-bacon-cheeseburger-sex-tape.

78 *"What unites the women":* Kim Chernin, *The Obsession: Reflections on the Tyranny of Slenderness* (New York: Harper Perennial, 1994), 101.

81 *"The pattern of the perfect body"*: Eve Ensler, *The Good Body* (New York: Villard, 2004), xii.

82 *"The choices we make"*: Oprah Winfrey, "What Are You Hungry For? Hint: It's Not Food," O, April 2010.

6. BEING A FASHIONISTA
CAN BE EMPOWERING

86 *"It's horrifying"*: Kate Schweitzer, "Tim Gunn's New Day Job," *Marie Claire*, December 2011.

87 *"If you want a girl"*: Quoted in Susan Faludi, *Backlash: The Undeclared War Against American Women*, fifteenth-anniversary edition (New York: Three Rivers Press, 2006), 185.

89 *"'Going soft'"*: Ibid., 196.
    1988 New York Times/CBS News poll: Ibid.

91 *"They're meant to be a kind of rejection"*: Lady Gaga, interview by Larry King, *Larry King Live*, CNN, June 1, 2010.

92 *"We want women to feel strong enough"*: James Montgomery, "Lady Gaga, Cyndi Lauper Raise AIDS Awareness with Lipstick," MTV .com, February 10, 2010, http://www.mtv.com/news/articles/1631673/ lady-gaga-cyndi-lauper-raise-aids-awareness-with-lipstick.jhtml.

94 *"That Madonna look was vulgar"*: quoted in Faludi, *Backlash*, 201.

98 *"I feel very strongly"*: Stacy London, as told to Andrea Bartz, "Sexy Feminist: Stacy London," December 3, 2007, http://sexyfeminist .com/2007/12/03/sexy-feminist-stacy-london/.

7. THE WORKING-WOMAN PROBLEM

100 *"playing the daffy and dependent girl"*: Susan Faludi, *Backlash: The Undeclared War Against American Women*, fifteenth-anniversary edition (1991; repr., New York: Three Rivers Press, 2006), 141.

101 *"women have flooded into the workplace"*: Nan Mooney, interview with the authors, December 2, 2011.
    30 Rock *hot-comic episode*: *30 Rock*, NBC, February 25, 2011.

102 *"My unsolicited advice to women"*: Tina Fey, *Bossypants* (Boston: Little, Brown, 2011), 144.

103 *Workplace Bullying Institute study*: Mickey Meece, "Backlash: Women Bullying Women at Work," *New York Times*, May 9, 2009.

104 *"Why help someone"*: Peggy Klaus, interview with the authors, June 21, 2011.
2006 Gallup Poll: http://www.gallup.com/poll/24346/americans-prefer -male-boss-female-boss.aspx.

107 *2011 White House report*: "Women in America: Indicators of Social and Economic Well-Being," Council on Women and Girls, http:// www.whitehouse.gov/administration/eop/cwg/data-on-women.

107 *19.6 million single-mom households*: Population Reference Bureau, http:// www.prb.org/Publications/PolicyBriefs/singlemotherfamilies.aspx.
most of Europe: Rebecca Ray, Janet C. Gornick, and John Schmitt, "Parental Leave Policies in 21 Countries," Center for Economic and Policy Research, September 2008.

108 *2008 National Science Foundation study*: Tamar Lewin, "Math Scores Show No Gap for Girls, Study Finds," *New York Times*, July 25, 2008.
Center for Work-Life Policy survey: Sylvia Ann Hewlett et al., "The Sponsor Effect," Center for Work-Life Policy, December 2010.

111 *"was a light in my life"*: Oprah Winfrey, "13 Memorable Cast Reunions," Oprah.com, May 6, 2011, http://www.oprah.com/oprahshow/ 13-Memorable-Cast-Reunions/.

8. BE A SEXY FEMINIST, NOT A SLUT-SHAMING ONE

117 *"Sexuality will always be"*: Lesley Rotchford, "Christina Aguilera Is All Woman," *Cosmopolitan*, October 2006, http://www.cosmopolitan .com/celebrity/exclusive/Christina-Aguilera-Is-All-Woman.

118 *"I think it's condescending"*: Amanda Hess, "Why Sex Positivity Is Bad for Feminism," *Sexist*, April 1, 2009, http://www.washingtoncitypaper .com/blogs/sexist/2009/04/01/why-sex-positivity-is-bad-for-feminism/.
"The whole argument": Ariel Levy, quoted in Kira Cochrane, "Thongs, Implants, and the Death of Real Fashion," *Guardian*, June 20, 2006.

119   *"Before it curdled"*: Maureen Dowd, "What's a Modern Girl to Do?," *New York Times*, October 30, 2005.

David Duchovny quote: Californication, Showtime, October 11, 2009.

details of Melissa Petro's background: Claire Gordon, "'Hooker Teacher' Forced to Resign, Now Can't Find Work," AOL.com, February 15, 2012.

120   *"Bronx Art Teacher"*: Bill Hutchinson, *New York Post*, September 28, 2010.

"As an advocate": Melissa Petro, "The 'Hooker Teacher' Tells All," Salon.com, May 4, 2011.

121   *some feminist groups promoted lesbian separatism*: Carolyn Bronstein, *Battling Pornography* (Cambridge: Cambridge University Press, 2011), 58.

"women who cut their ties": Charlotte Bunch, "Lesbians in Revolt," *Furies* 1 (January 1972): 8–9.

"bring their ideals about integrity": Lillian Faderman, *Odd Girls and Twilight Lovers* (pbk.; New York: Penguin, 1992), 220.

Florida's Pagoda: Sarah Kershaw, "My Sister's Keeper," *New York Times*, January 30, 2009.

122   *"Pornography is the theory"*: Robin Morgan, *Going Too Far* (New York: Vintage Books, 1978), 169.

"I am opposed": Diana Russell, e-mail interview with the authors, September 1, 2011.

Q&A with Melissa Broudo: Melissa Broudo, e-mail interview with the authors, August 22, 2011.

125   *"A good deal of current feminist literature"*: Gayle S. Rubin, *Deviations* (Durham, NC: Duke University Press, 2011), 137.

127   *Sarah Katherine Lewis's piece on stripping*: Sarah Katherine Lewis, "Is Stripping a Feminist Act?," Alternet.com, May 4, 2007.

128   *"giving intellectual pretensions"*: Maureen Dowd, "How to Snag 2,000 Men," *New York Times*, July 2, 1997.

129   *"The war between the sexes is over"*: *Crazy, Stupid, Love* (Warner Bros., 2011).

9. FLIRTING AND DATING

135 *Naomi Wolf quote*: Naomi Wolf, new introduction to *The Beauty Myth: How Images of Beauty Are Used Against Women* (1991; repr., New York: Harper Perennial, 2002), 177.

140 *Suzanne Venker quote*: Paul Bedard, "5 Ways Feminism Has Ruined America," USNews.com, March 4, 2011.

141 *"A woman's sense of self"*: John Gray, *Men Are from Mars, Women Are from Venus* (New York: HarperCollins, 1992), 12.

142 *"Just as a man is fulfilled"*: Ibid., 36.
  Naomi Weisstein quote: Naomi Weisstein, "Woman as Nigger," *Psychology Today* 3 (October 1969).
  "Let us return": Naomi Weisstein, "Power, Resistance, and Science," *Feminism and Psychology* 3 (June 1993): 239–45.

143 *"It's about giving ourselves"*: Pamela Haag, interview with the authors, November 17, 2011.

10. FEMINISM IN THE BEDROOM

147 *"There's this idea"*: "Sexy Feminists Read: Jaclyn Friedman's *What You Really Really Want*," *Sexy Feminist*, December 6, 2011, http://sexyfeminist.com/2011/12/06/sexy-feminists-read-jaclyn-friedmans-what-you-really-really-want/.
  "Most women prefer": Courtney Hutchison, "Feminism as the Anti-Viagra," ABCNews.com, April 18, 2011.

148 *"best way to make your sex life more egalitarian"*: "Sexy Feminists Read: Jaclyn Friedman."

149 *"voluntary motherhood"*: Betty A. DeBerg, *Ungodly Women* (Atlanta: Mercer University Press, 2000), 36.
  birth control origins: Margaret Sanger Papers Project, New York University, http://www.nyu.edu/projects/sanger/secure/aboutms/index.html.
  first family-planning clinic: Estelle B. Freedman, *The Essential Feminist Reader* (New York: Random House, 2007), 211.
  Guttmacher Institute study: http://www.guttmacher.org/media/nr/2011/04/13/index.html.

150 *hundred million women:* Nancy Gibbs, "The Pill at 50," *Time*, April 22, 2010.

151 *Plan B restrictions:* Irin Carmon, "Obama Says No to Plan B for Teens," Salon.com, December 7, 2011.
FDA warning on Yaz and Yasmin: http://www.fda.gov/Safety/Med-Watch/SafetyInformation/SafetyAlertsforHumanMedicalProducts/ucm299605.htm?source=govdelivery.

152 *CDC statistics on birth control effectiveness:* http://www.cdc.gov/reproductivehealth/unintendedpregnancy/contraception.htm.
Griswold v. Connecticut: *Congressional Record*, June 7, 2005, 11698.

153 *$15 to $50 per month:* Maggie Mahar, "Why Free Birth Control Will Not Hike the Cost of Your Insurance," Time.com, February 14, 2012.

154 *condom history:* Daniel DeNoon, "Birth Control Timeline," WebMD.com, July 17, 2003.
birth control pill approved: "American Experience: The Pill," PBS.org, http://www.pbs.org/wgbh/amex/pill/timeline/timeline2.html.
first hormone shot: K. Aleisha Fetters, "Spotlight: Birth Control," Womenshealth.com, http://www.womenshealthmag.com/health/history-of-birth-control-0.

155 *first emergency contraception:* "FDA Approves First Emergency Contraception Kit," CNN.com, September 2, 1998.
first continuous birth control pill: Katherine Kam, "No More Periods," WebMD.com, http://www.webmd.com/sex/birth-control/features/no-more-periods.
"war on women's health": Sarah Bibi, "6,000 Rally to Stop 'War on Women's Health,'" Gothamist.com, February 27, 2011.

156 *"The argument that women who enjoy BDSM":* Megan Carpentier, "BDSM and Feminism," Jezebel.com, October 17, 2010.
"I think that sexuality": "Sexy Feminists Read: Jaclyn Friedman."

157 *"rape fantasies are fine":* Ibid.

159 *study by Terri Fisher:* Katie Moisse, "Men Think About Sex, Just Not Non-Stop," ABCNews.com, November 29, 2011.

11. FEMINIST RELATIONSHIPS

165 *Betty Friedan's relationship with husband:* Marcia Cohen, "Books: Carl Friedan Strikes Back," *New York,* May 29, 2000.

166 *Jessica Valenti on her wedding:* Jessica Valenti, "My Big Feminist Wedding," *Guardian,* April 23, 2009.

173 *divorce rate has fallen:* Tara Parker-Pope, "She Works. They're Happy," *New York Times,* January 22, 2010.

    housework-sex link: Sue Shellenbarger, "Does More Housework Mean More Sex?," *Juggle,* October 21, 2009.

    partnerships in which woman outranks man: Pew Research Center, "Women, Men, and the New Economics of Marriage," January 19, 2010.

174 *"There are relationships":* "Sexy Feminists Read: *The Guy's Guide to Feminism,*" *Sexy Feminist,* December 12, 2011, http://sexyfeminist .com/2011/12/12/sexy-feminists-read-the-guys-guide-to-feminism/.

    "I clean the house": Ani DiFranco, quoted in Jennifer Baumgardner, *F'em* (Berkeley, CA: Seal Press, 2011), 148.

178 *"a perfect type of marriage":* "Sexy Feminists Read: Pamela Haag's *Marriage Confidential,*" *Sexy Feminist,* November 17, 2011, http:// sexyfeminist.com/2011/11/17/sexy-feminists-read-pamela-haags -marriage-confidential/.

180 *statistics on name changes and history of Lucy Stone:* Lucy Stone League, http://www.lucystoneleague.org/.

12. FEMALE FRIENDSHIP

185 *Mary Wollstonecraft's friendships:* Chawton House Library biography of Wollstonecraft, http://www.chawtonhouse.org/library/biographies/ wollstonecraft.html.

    Wollstonecraft's letter to Jane Arden: Janet Todd, *The Collected Letters of Mary Wollstonecraft* (New York: Columbia University Press, 2003), 16.

186 *"By blaring the hetero-relational message":* Janice Raymond, *A Passion for Friends,* 2nd ed. (1986; repr., Melbourne, Australia: Spinifex Press, 2001), 151.

"*I've always been attracted to*": Jennifer Baumgardner, personal interview with the authors, January 5, 2012.

"*I think there is something*": Amy Richards, personal interview with the authors, January 5, 2012.

188   "*We women swim in shark-infested waters*": Kelly Valen, "My Sorority Pledge? I Swore Off Sisterhood," *New York Times*, December 2, 2007.

190   "*She's done so many things*": Allison, personal interviews with the authors, October 2011.

AFTERWORD: ACTIVISM IS SEXY

199   "*personhood movement*": Irin Carmon, "Personhood, the Undead Movement, Marches On," Salon.com, March 27, 2012.

200   *80 percent of anti-choice Americans*: Priya Jain, "The Battle to Ban Birth Control," Salon.com, March 20, 2006.

202   *teen mentoring statistics*: National Mentoring Partnership, http://www.mentoring.org.

203   *Haiti earthquake statistics*: "Haiti Lies in Ruins; Grim Search for Untold Dead," *New York Times*, January 13, 2010.

     Bangladesh statistics: BBC News, November 19, 2007, http://news.bbc.co.uk/2/hi/south_asia/7100957.stm; World Hunger Organization, http://www.worldhunger.org.

207   *selective abortions*: David Brown, "Sex-Selective Abortions on Rise in India Among Couples Without Boys," *Washington Post*, May 23, 2011.

     65 million girls are out of school: UNICEF 2010 State of the World's Children Report, http://www.unicef.org.

208   *leading cause of injury and death*: "Facts about Violence," http://www.feminist.com/antiviolence/facts.html.

209   *Sexual-violence statistics*: RAINN, http://www.rainn.org; Domestic Violence Resource Center, http://http://www.dvrc-or.org.

     More than thirty million people: Not for Sale Campaign, http://www.notforsalecampaign.org/about/slavery/.

ACKNOWLEDGMENTS

No one truly writes a book alone, and in this case, no one truly writes a book as just two people either. We must thank the following people: Charles Salzberg, for fostering our feminist publishing dreams from the start; Sally Koslow, for being a great role model; the writers who have helped keep our website vital since its inception, especially the prolific Allison Hantschel and A. K. Whitney; our life partners, Jesse Davis and Ken Rudúlph, for debating the issues with us, editing us, questioning us, and being the sexiest male feminists we know; our families, for making us the feminists we are; Laurie Abkemeier, our agent, our role model, the woman who made our dreams come true; our tough manuscript editing team, including Wendy Thomas Russell and Erin Mahoney Harris; our editor Nicole Angeloro; and our personal feminist icons Jennifer Baumgardner, Susan Faludi, Amy Richards, Gloria Steinem, Naomi Wolf, and the countless young feminists writing, rallying, and blogging today with the guts to own the label, preach the verse, and draw attention to the important things that matter to women. Special thanks to everyone who has read our labor of love, SexyFeminist.com. We definitely couldn't have done this without you.